II/s
7/06

NAIL STYLE

beautiful nails for every occasion

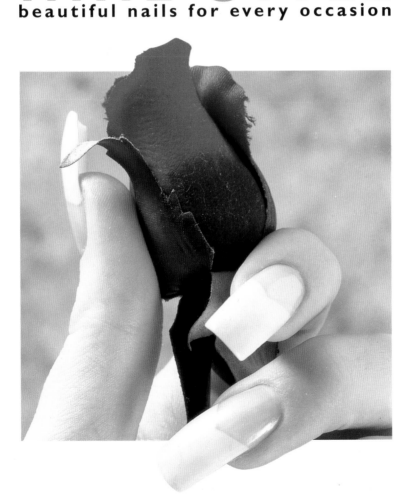

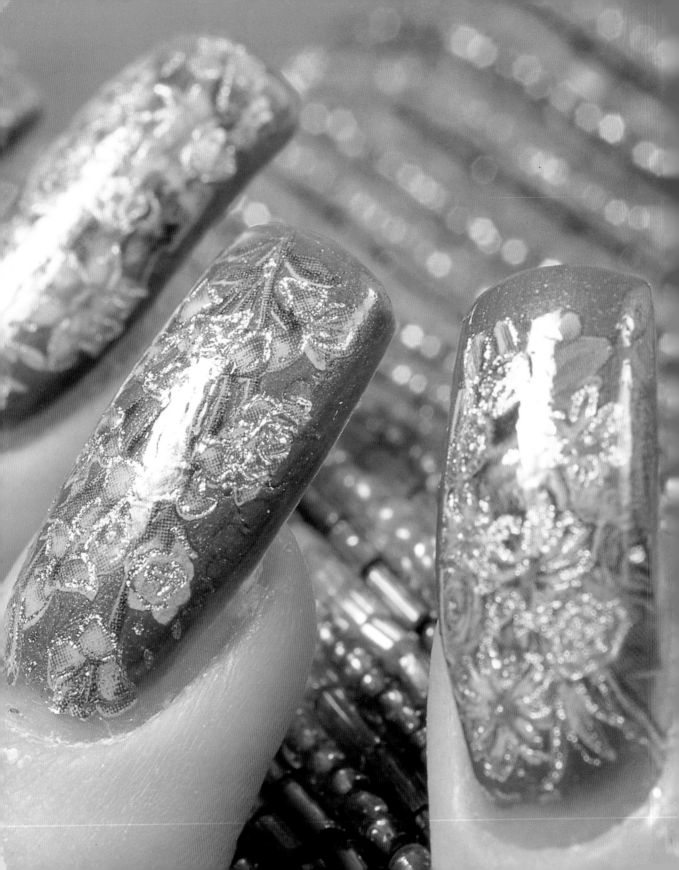

NAIL STYLE

beautiful nails for every occasion

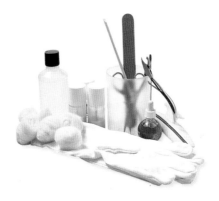

MARIE MINGAY

Sterling Publishing Co., Inc.
New York

Library of Congress Cataloging-in-Publication Data Available

2 4 6 8 10 9 7 5 3 1

Published in this edition in 2005 by Sterling Publishing Co., Inc.
387 Park Avenue South, New York, NY 10016

© 2000 D&S Books Limited

Distributed in Canada by Sterling Publishing
c/o Canadian Manda Group, 165 Dufferin Street
Toronto, Ontario, Canada M6K 3H6

Every effort has been made to ensure that all the information in this book is accurate. However, due to differing conditions, tools, and individual skills, the publisher cannot be responsible for any injuries, losses, and other damages which may result from the use of the information in this book.

Editorial Director: Sarah King
Editor: Clare Haworth-Maden
Project Editor: Sarah Harris
Photographer: Paul Forrester
Designer: Axis Design Editions Limited

Printed in China
All rights reserved

ISBN 1-4027-2027-0

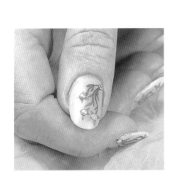

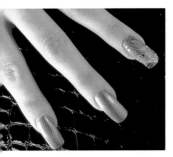

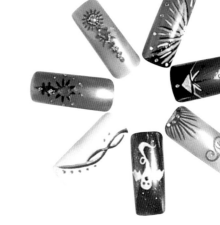

Contents

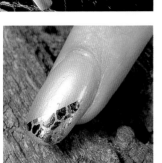

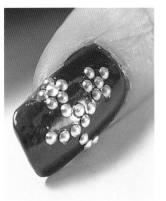

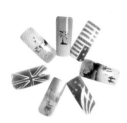

Introduction

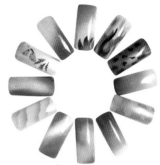

While traveling around the world over the years, I have found that having beautiful nails boosts my confidence. Unfortunately, the majority of people find maintaining a manicured look very difficult, and just when you think that your nails are looking their best, you usually break one.

Nail art can provide a delicate, romantic finish to your appearance – particularly important on special occasions.

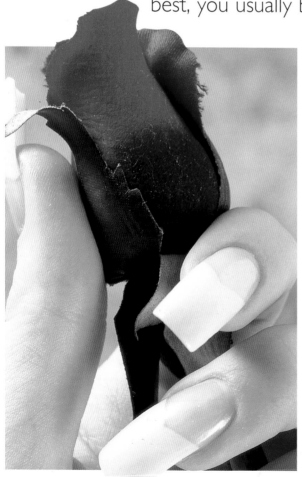

Creating lovely nails is the largest growth area of the beauty business. Nail art, airbrushing, and designer nail jewelry generate huge sales, not only in the world's beauty salons and nail bars, but also in less specialised stores, like drug stores. You can go back to the 1970s by transforming your nails with holographic and glittering acrylics, with nail extensions that often have fabulous names, like "Staying Alive," "Foxy Lady," "Funky Town," "Shake Your Groovy Thing," and "Disco Nights." You can also design and create your own holographic pictures to add to nail extensions, which can be adorned with nail jewelry made from 14-karat or white gold, silver, and all sorts of gems – including diamonds – in any color you like, while airbrushing, decals (picture transfers), and rhinestones can make up any number of shapes and designs. I shall not only advise you on general nail shapes, but also on designs that will complement your hands, giving you greater confidence in your appearance.

Our nails are complicated structures, which, like hair and skin, need moisturizing and protecting from the damage that the day-to-day environment, as well as the elements, may cause. In many cases, nails require treatments and maintenance

A proper nailcare routine is essential before you apply any nail art.

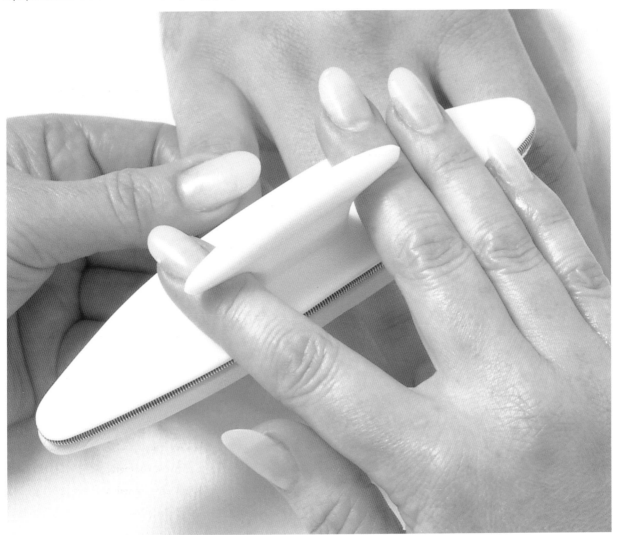

programs, and sometimes even a doctor's prescription. I hope that this book will give you a better understanding of the everyday problems that can affect nails, along with a basic knowledge of the specialized treatments that you can request from a nail technician or manicurist.

There are many reasons why some people prefer natural nailcare, and a number of comprehensive, professional treatments and nailcare ranges are today available to deal with any problem. Because everyone's nails are completely different, they should be given an individual assessment and maintained with a program that suits them best. This book will provide advice on doing so.

Beautiful nails – be they natural or extended, airbrushed or jeweled – are at your fingertips. Let your only restriction be your imagination, and let's start creating.

Nailcare Equipment and Materials

Caring for your nails is vital if you are to achieve a beautiful finish for your nail art. There are several products which you will need in order to maintain healthy nails.

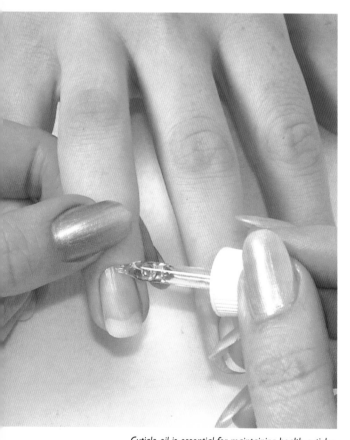

Cuticle oil is essential for maintaining health cuticles.

Cuticle Conditioners ✓

Cuticle conditioners and creams will keep your cuticles soft and easy to care for. For the maximum benefit, use them at night to achieve the best results.

Cuticle Removers ✓

Cuticle removers are used to loosen and lift off any excess, dry cuticle from the nail plate, which, if left, can have an overlapping and encroaching effect on the nail, causing it to harden and dry, and ultimately to become damaged.

Hand Creams and Nail Moisturisers

Hand creams and nail moisturisers are a must (see Natural manicure, page 22). It is always advisable to purchase ones that contain an ultraviolet (U.V.) filter, as well as a water-based emulsion cream suitable for everyday use. You can buy hand creams that condition your nails, too, which may come as a surprise until you realize that because 18 percent of your nails are made up of water, they can become dehydrated, just like your skin and body.

Moisturizing your hands will keep them soft, and helps ensure healthy nails.

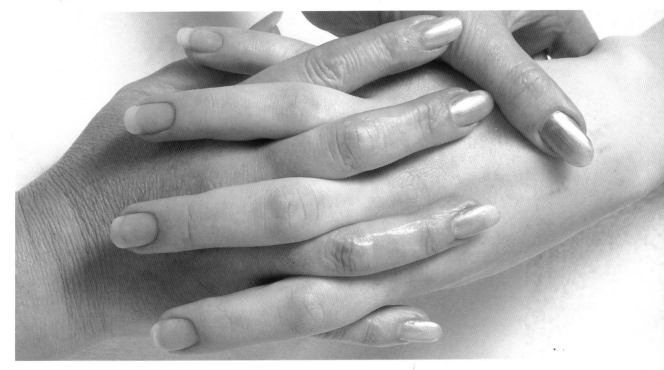

Give yourself a specialized treatment by using an intensive hand cream at night, which will have a deep-acting, moisturizing effect. To reap the greatest benefits, put on cotton gloves after applying it to achieve maximum moisture retention.

Emery Boards

Never use a metal nail file – emery boards cause far less damage. Like sandpaper, emery boards come in various grades denoting different levels of coarseness. Unless your nails are extremely strong, it is usually best to use a fine-graded emery board which will not damage the nail.

Nail Blocks

White nail blocks are used to remove the natural sheen from your nails, to reduce any ridges that are in the early stages of development, and to smooth the nail surface.

Nail Buffers

Nail buffers are sold in various styles, such as four-sided or chamois-leather buffers. Buffing your nails is a great way to stimulate the blood flow within your nail plate. It also gives your nails a natural, mirrorlike sheen.

White Nail Pencils

A great way to cheat, using a white nail pencil can conceal discoloration at the tip of the nail and give it a much cleaner look. To get the maximum benefit from your white pencil, wet the tip and gently rub it underneath the nail tip. You can also buy nail brighteners, which contain nail conditioners, as well as gentle,

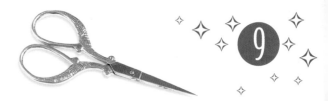

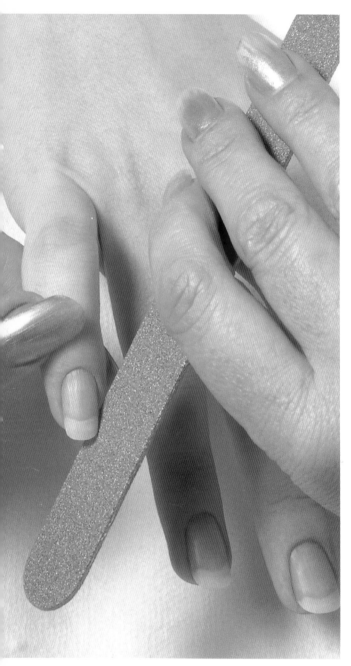

natural bleaching agents. An example is lemon juice, which you can add to a bowl of water before soaking your hands for a few minutes.

Nail Hardeners and Strengtheners

A number of products combine nail hardeners and strengtheners with either a base or topcoat. Some have been made to a specific formula, for example, those that contain various levels of protein to treat weak, flaking nails or dry, brittle nails. If you are unsure which is best suited to your nails, seek professional advice from a nail technician or manicurist. Never apply the product too close to the cuticle or surrounding finger edges, which will only cause dryness and sometimes more serious problems. Always read the instructions on the packet and follow them implicitly.

Oils

Oils that treat and feed nails come in many forms. Manicurists usually recommend that you use them nightly to condition your nails and promote growth. They can also help to prevent unsightly cracks developing around the sides of the nails, which may cause hang nails. A further benefit is that they condition your cuticles, as well as your nails. And last, but not least, they precondition the new part of the nail that you cannot see.

Orange sticks

Orange sticks are generally used for pushing back softened cuticles and cleaning under nails. Always attach a small amount of absorbent cotton to the orange stick to make it a gentler tool (although nail technicians usually use a metal implement, they have been professionally trained). Orange sticks are useful accessories when creating nail art, and can also be used as corrector pens if you do not have the real thing to hand.

Always use an emery board to file your nails. A metal file will cause far more damage.

False Nails

False nails, which cover the entire nail plate, come in many shapes, designs, and forms, including airbrushed, French polished, square-finished, and curve-tipped nails. They are normally secured by either double-sided, sticky backs or nail glue. You will have to size up each of your nails in turn before securing false nails. Using such nail extensions is only recommended on a short-term basis, perhaps for a special occasion or if you have broken a nail and need to protect it, because wearing a false nail over the long term will damage the nail if it is not removed properly. Never remove a false nail with anything other than the correct solvent. If in doubt, seek professional advice.

Nail Scissors and Clippers

You will not necessarily need nail scissors if you manicure your nails regularly. If you do use nail scissors, however, always cut your nails when they are hard, and not when you have soaked them in warm water, which will cause them to split. The same advice applies to nail clippers.

Toe Separators and Pedicure Pads

Toe separators and pedicure pads are really useful tools and offer a quick and easy way of ensuring that you do not smudge your toenail enamel. They also make enamel easier to apply.

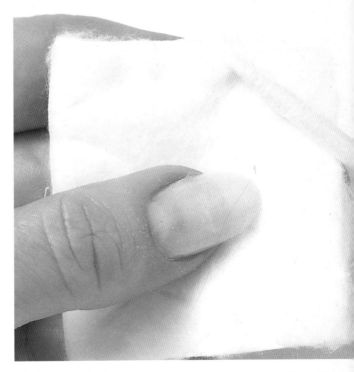

Applying some absorbent cotton to an orange stick will make it gentler to use.

Alternatively, you could weave a tissue in and out between your toes. Absorbent-cotton balls are not recommended, because they may shed fluff on your beautifully painted toenails. Walking while wearing pedicure pads is a great exercise for your feet and toes, and will help keep joints flexible.

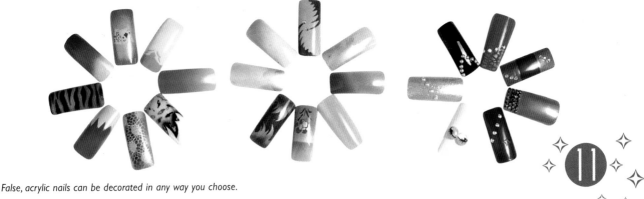

False, acrylic nails can be decorated in any way you choose.

Base Coats

You will need to prepare your canvas properly if you want to maximize the impact of any form of nail art, from the simplest of enamels to more outrageous designs. A base coat (or, in the case of airbrushing, a foundation coat) primes the nail surface before you work on it. It will also stop nails from becoming stained, which sometimes happens when dark colors have been used. Some base coats contain protein-based, nail-hardening ingredients. Remember to apply a base coat every time you paint or decorate your nails.

Topcoats

Topcoats are a great asset, in that they complete the finishing touch and give nails a smooth, glassy sheen and an ultraglossy shine. They protect the nail enamel from chipping, while a number reduce the potential yellowing of a French manicure and also incorporate a protein base that will condition your nails. Some contain a U.V. screen, which is only recommended for use on natural nails and not on colored enamel, because it will undermine the color.

Professional tip: *applying another coat of topcoat as a middle stage in your manicure or nail art will give it renewed sparkle.*

Nail Extensions

Permagloss is a gel extension that is used over acrylic nails, giving a high-density, gloss finish and added protection. It contains a U.V.-light-resistant substance and a sealant.

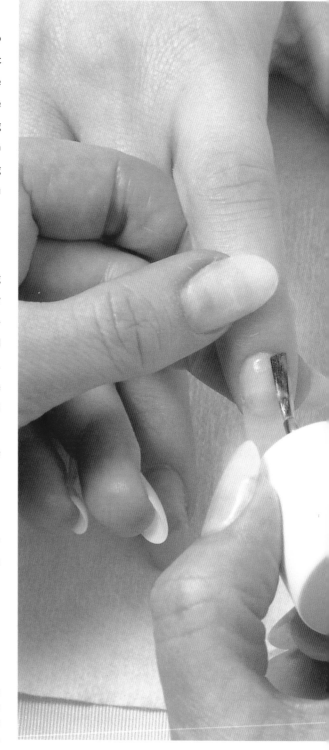

Base coats are essential to prepare your nail for any type of nail art.

Caring for Your Nails

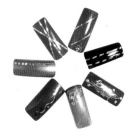

Like your hair and skin, your nails will suffer if you are not in good health or are stressed. It is important that your diet is good, that you exercise, and that you get plenty of fresh air. Taking vitamin supplements, resting, and sleeping well will all help your nails, too. Interestingly, nails grow faster in warmer climates (or in summer) than in cold ones (or in winter).

Getting the Balance Right

In the majority of cases, the shape and strength of your nails is due to the genetic factors that you have inherited from either of your parents. If there were a recipe to promote the hardest possible nails, it would consist of vitamins and minerals, particularly vitamin A, calcium and iodine (which strengthens nails, reduces splitting and promotes growth). Nail-friendly foods include dairy products, fish, shellfish, fresh vegetables (especially broccoli and spinach) and fruit – particularly kiwi. A lack of biotin (a member of the vitamin B family) in the body can cause brittle nails, and tomatoes, apricots, carrots and cherries can help to rectify this deficiency. Other foods that are rich in biotin are peanut butter, sesame seeds, wholegrains, liver and eggs.

You can take steps to combat such problems as nail deformation (unsightly ridges that often occur after a serious illness) by eating sunflower seeds, walnuts and rye bread every day. It

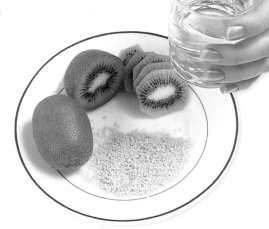

A healthy diet is essential for maintaining healthy nails.

will take from three to six months before you see any change in the condition of your nail, however, so don't expect an immediate improvement. Having a professional manicure will also help considerably. In addition, you could take a vitamin called combination K (an organic-tissue salt stocked by most health stores), which will promote nail, as well as hair, growth. Again, however, it will take up to six months before you see the beneficial effect of taking this supplement.

Hand Creams and Nail Conditioners

Condition your nails in the same way you condition your hair and moisturize your skin (and this applies just as much to men as to women). Just as you opt for the conditioner or moisturizer that suits your hair or skin type best, when choosing a hand cream or nail conditioner remember that everyone's nails have different needs.

It is important that you appreciate that if you use only an ordinary, everyday hand cream, your hands and nails will miss out on the benefits offered by intensive hand treatments, cuticle oils, or creams. It is best to use an intensive hand cream at night and an ordinary hand cream throughout the day.

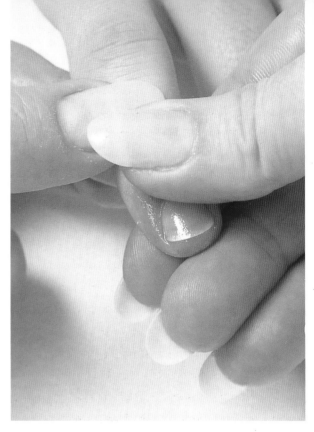

Creams and oils are vital for conditioning your nails.

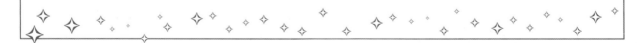

Determining the Best Nail Shape to Complement Your Hands

Small, dainty hands usually look best if the nails are short and slightly oval. A pale shade of nail enamel complements the shape well.

✦

Oval-shaped hands suit more vibrant colors.

✦

Medium-sized to broad hands often have wider nails, which look best when they are of a moderate length and are slightly pointed. Painting the nails with a dark enamel, and leaving a narrow, unvarnished edge at each side, makes them appear longer and slimmer.

✦

Large, square hands typically have large, square nails, which should be filed to a point (try to follow the shape of your fingertips). When painting them, leave a thin, unvarnished line on each side of the nail. Remember that darker colors usually give a more dramatic look.

Try to have a professional manicure at least once a month, which will keep your hands and nails in optimum condition. If you are worried about nail infections or any other nail problems, seek the advice of your nail technician – trawling through the overwhelming choice on the drug-store's shelves will probably leave you feeling confused.

Hand Massages

Hands are one of the first parts of the body to show age, so it is important to look after them by following a regular hand- and nailcare regime. Although well-groomed nails and smooth hands were once considered the preserve of the "idle rich," today we are more aware of our hands' appearance. Displaying your hands, rather than feeling that you have to hide them away, is a real confidence-booster, and it's amazing how many people comment on lovely hands and nails. Massages and manicures are treatments that you can perform yourself with only a little effort, and once you've started your new regime you won't want to stop.

A hand massage should be an integral part of your nailcare routine.

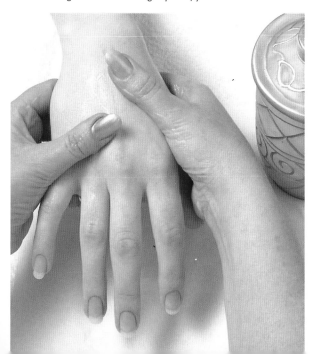

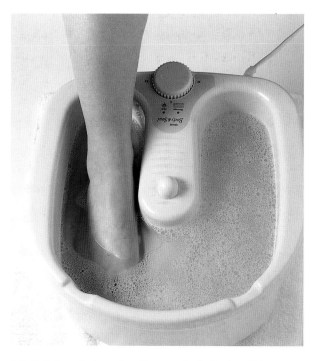

A footbath is a relaxing and soothing way of refreshing your feet.

Pedicure

The feet are probably the most neglected area of the body in most people's beauty regime, in spite of the extremely hard work they do each day. Not only do they support the whole weight of the body day in and day out, but the localized pressure concentrates to the equivalent of as much as three times the total body weight in key areas. Even without the added pressure created when you walk, this is why the skin on the feet can be up to seven times thicker than the skin on the rest of the body.

A regular pedicure routine can help refresh and revitalize the feet, as well as helping to prevent or minimize foot problems. A regular soak in warm water – which can be scented with aromatherapy oils if you wish – can be a soothing and relaxing start to your pedicure. A special foot bath or spa is an enjoyable treat, but a bowl of water is just as effective.

Knowing Your Nail Cosmetics

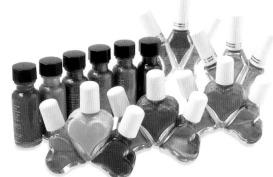

A wide range of nail enamel is available, from subtle, pastel colors to outrageously bright, vibrant colors, varying in price from as little as a few dollars per bottle to many dollars more. If you are ambitious, you could try to mix different enamels to create your own colors. New types of nail enamel are constantly hitting the shelves, including enamel that glows in the dark, fluorescent and neon enamels, clear enamel that contains suspended dots or strands of glitter in many colors, mood-tone enamels, and crackle-glaze enamels. You can even buy nail enamel that smells of fruit, whose fragrance lasts for three to four days. And with the advent of nail-art kits, the choice is growing ever larger. The following are just a few examples of special types of nail enamel available.

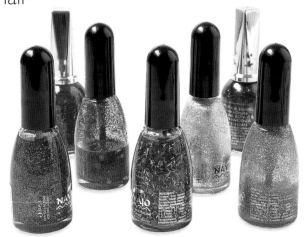

Glitter enamels are just some of the special-effect enamels available.

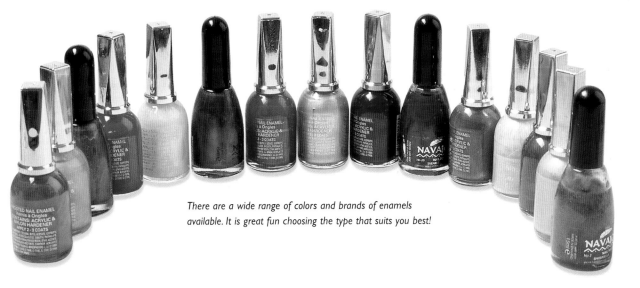

There are a wide range of colors and brands of enamels available. It is great fun choosing the type that suits you best!

Mood-tone Enamels

Mood-tone enamels are a new and exciting range of products that respond to your body heat or mood. They are available in a number of colors, from pastels to funkier, stronger hues, with either a glittering or a smooth finish. The colder you are, the darker the color will become, and as your body warms up the color lightens. It is fascinating to watch the colors change, particularly when the cuticle area is lighter and the tip of the nail is dark (like a French polish in reverse). If you are daring, you could combine mood-tone enamels.

Light-variation Enamels

Light-variation enamels are metallic-based substances that vary in color from light to dark shades. They change their tone according to the light; for example, a gold light-variation polish will change from gold to copper, and from copper to coppery pink, and then a copper-kettle tone, depending on whether it is night or day or if you are in strong sunlight. In common with any other enamel, always paint a base coat under them. You will probably need to use two to three coats for maximum effect.

Fruity Enamels

Sweet-smelling, fruity enamels – which include strawberry, blackberry, blueberry, kiwi, lime, and apricot – have a glittery shimmer. They can either have their own color definition or can be painted over another nail enamel to give variation in color. If you use a blueberry base nail enamel under a blueberry fruity enamel, a deep-eggplant color will result. You could also be a little more creative and apply fruity enamel either diagonally across the nail or along the center for a completely different look that has a lovely scent. The scent will last for approximately four days, depending on your body temperature and the prevailing climate.

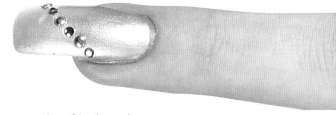

Beautiful nail enamel can be enhanced with creative nail art.

17

Nowadays, the packaging of nail enamels is almost as important as the enamel inside!

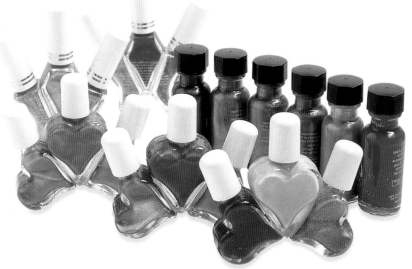

Crackle-glaze Enamels

Crackle-glaze nail enamels give a broken, shattered effect when painted over your base nail enamel. They can also change the depth and tone of color of your base nail enamel. They look better painted over darker colors rather than over pale or pastel ones, as this reflects more.

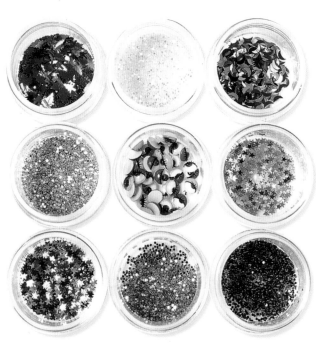

As well as enamels, there is a range of accessories available to liven up your nails. These will be covered in more detail in the projects

Opalescent Paints

Opalescent paints, which come in six colors, offer an exciting way of creating a different look. They look best when painted over darker shades, giving them greater depth and definition. You will need special tools when working with opalescent paints (see Chapter 7).

Acrylic Paints

With practice you can create some amazing designs with acrylic paints, which are sold in a wide range of colors. You will need special tools for applying them.

Getting the Best out of Nail Enamels

When buying a nail enamel, choose a smaller, rather than a larger, bottle, as nail enamels have a limited shelf life. It is best to store nail enamels in the refrigerator, or at the very least out of direct sunlight and away from a heat source.

Bottles of nail enamel contain a small, stainless-steel ball, which helps you to mix the color to a smooth and uniform consistency. Mix nail enamel by turning the bottle upside down and rolling it between your hands, which will act to prevent air bubbles forming.

There is no need to break your nails when opening old or tight-topped bottles of nail enamel. Smear a little petroleum jelly around the neck of the bottle or hold it under hot water.

Nail-enamel Thinners

Nail-enamel thinners are mainly used when nail polish has become slightly thick, giving colors a longer shelf-life. Make sure that you buy products that are clearly labeled as being nail-enamel thinners and never confuse them with nail-enamel removers or paint thinners (which have a completely different chemical structure), both of which will damage the structure of your nail enamel, not to mention your nails.

Nail-enamel Removers

Nail-enamel removers are sold in various forms: in bottles, as ready-infused pads, or as jars that contain a sponge with a hole in the center. Always use an acetone-free nail-enamel remover, which will help to reduce dryness and prevent your nails from becoming brittle and your cuticles from dehydrating. Always wash your hands after using a nail-enamel remover.

Professional Tip:

Always roll the bottle (never shake it) between your hands to prevent any blobbing. Starting from the cuticle, apply the enamel using only two to three strokes to give a smooth finish. Most nail enamels require two to three coats before you attain a true color. In order to ensure that you don't smudge your nail enamel, always use a quick-drying topcoat.

Repairing a Smudged Nail

Despite all your best efforts, it is very easy to smudge your nail enamel, whether by catching it on something, or not allowing coats to dry thoroughly between applications. Unless you have smeared the whole nail, in which case your best bet is to clean the nail and start again, you can make minor repairs very quickly and easily.

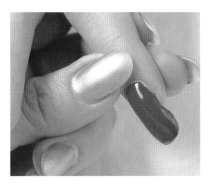

1 This is the kind of smear you are likely to get quite easily.

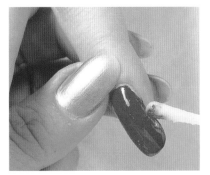

2 Dip a cotton bud in nail-enamel remover, so that it is moist, but not soaking wet. Gently smooth over the smear.

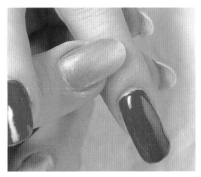

3 Unless the damage is too great, your nail will be as good as new!

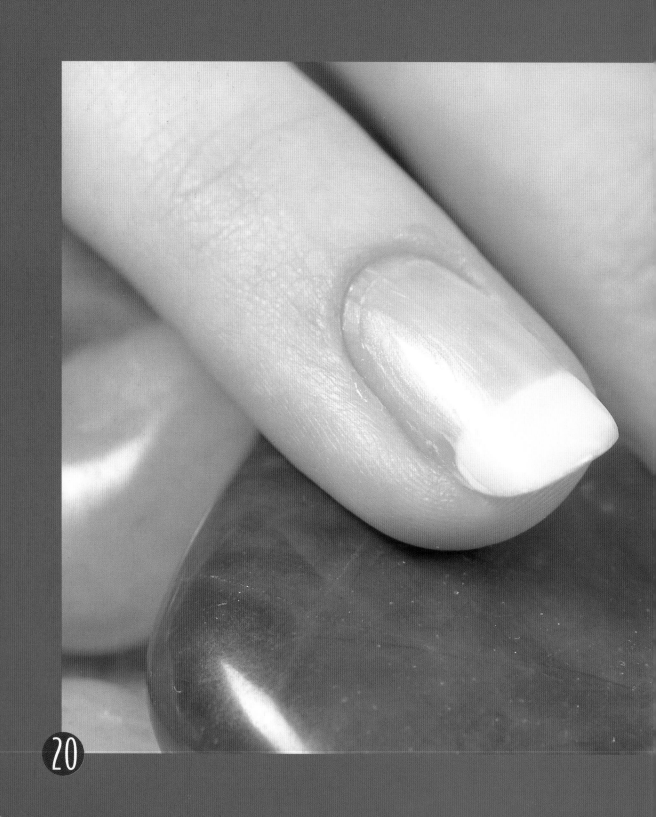

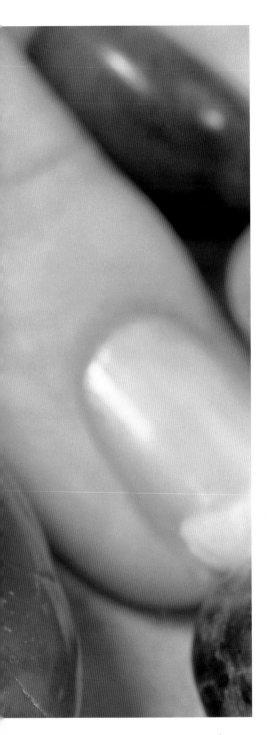

Basic Nailcare and Effects

We have already looked at the importance of caring for your nails in order to make them the best possible canvas for your nail art. This chapter looks at some simple and effective nailcare techniques, as well as some basic enamel effects that will give your nails an extra lift.

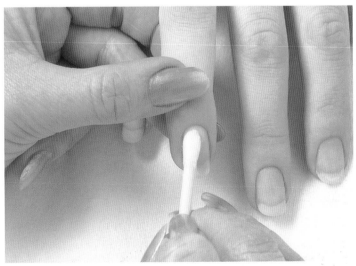

Natural Manicure

Having decided on your nail art – be it elegantly simple or totally outrageous – you will have to prepare your nails before applying it, much as an artist prepares a canvas before embarking on a work of art.

You Will Need

Finest-grain emery board

❖

Cuticle-removing oil or cream

❖

Warm water containing an essential oil

❖

Soft towel

❖

Orange stick

❖

Absorbent cotton or pads

❖

Cuticle trimmers

❖

Nail-buffing block

❖

Treatment hand cream

❖

Cotton gloves

❖

Base coat

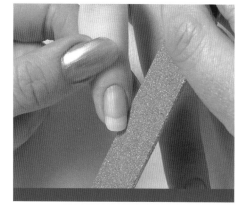

1 First remove any jewelry. Curl your fingers over and hold a finest-grain emery board at an angle to each nail in turn. File in one direction only, using a sweeping action, and do not file in a back-and-forth direction. Working from the sides to the middle of the nail tip, aim for a slightly square shape, and file down into your side walls (nail edges).

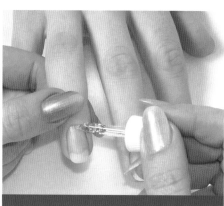

2 Apply a generous amount of cuticle-remover cream or oil, massaging it in around the cuticles using circular movements.

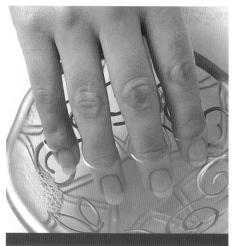

3 Soak your nails in warm water for at least five minutes.

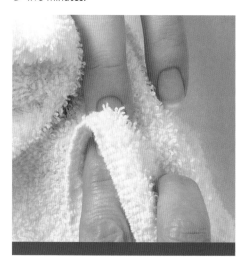

4 Dry your hands thoroughly with a soft towel. You now need to gently push back your softened cuticles.

22

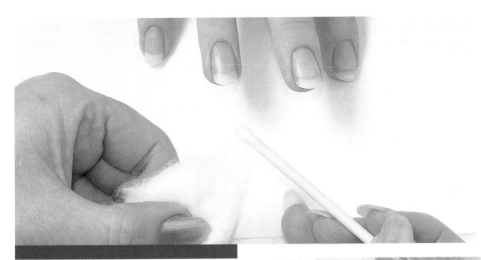

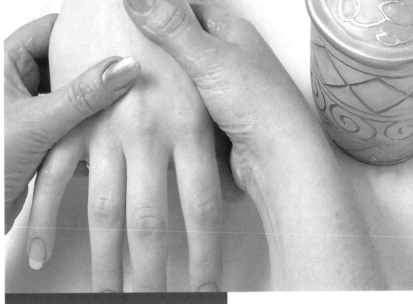

5 An ordinary cotton bud is not adequate for this, but you can make your own using an orange stick and an absorbent cotton pad. Wrap the tip of the orange stick in a few strands of cotton from the pad.

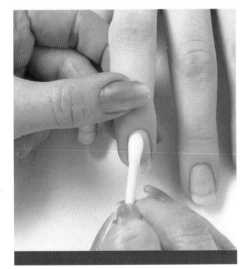

6 While your cuticles are still soft, gently push them back either with the orange stick, or you can use your finger, wrapped in a soft towel (you could also do this after a bath.) You may need to trim your cuticles with a cuticle trimmer, but regard this as a last resort, and if you do it yourself take the utmost care. This procedure should really be left to a nail technician, because if the cuticle is cut too low it may become infected.

7 Now that you've completed the first stages of your manicure, give yourself a hand massage (see page 28).

8 Remove any excess cream or oil from your nails with warm, soapy water and absorbent cotton or an absorbent-cotton pad. If the oil or cream were left, it would react with your nail enamel and ruin your nail art.

9 Apply a base coat to your nails. This will form the "canvas" for your nail art.

23

Male Manicure

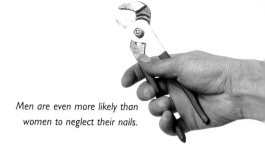

Men are even more likely than women to neglect their nails.

One of the most sweeping changes in recent years is that men are becoming more aware of their grooming, not just their hair and skin, but also their hands and feet. Pampering the body, and manicures in particular, were not regarded as macho, but a good hand and nail program is tremendously relaxing and the results can give you that extra edge and confidence needed to tackle the challenges of the fast-moving world in which we live today.

You Will Need

Finest-grain emery board

✧

Cuticle-removing oil or cream

✧

Warm water containing an essential oil

✧

Soft towel

✧

Orange stick

✧

Absorbent cotton

✧

Cuticle trimmers

✧

Nail-buffing block

✧

Treatment hand cream

✧

Cotton gloves

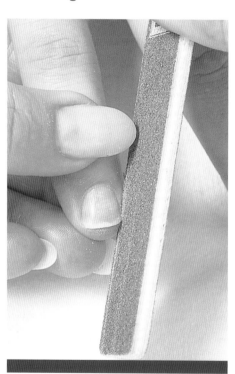

1 First you must file the nails into shape with an emery board. Never use a rough sawing motion – always file in the same direction. First file across the top of the nail.

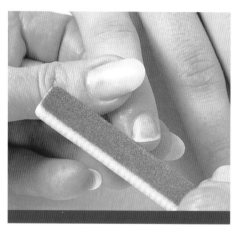

2 Now file down the sides of the nail, again moving in one direction only.

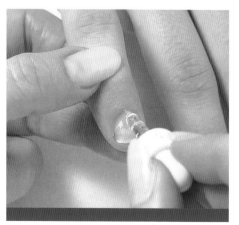

3 Place a few drops of cuticle oil on the cuticle of the first nail.

24

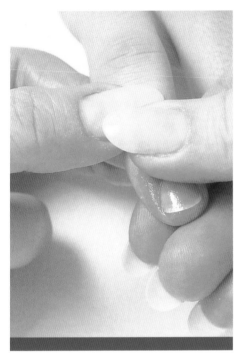

4 Gently massage the oil into the cuticle, making sure you cover the whole area.

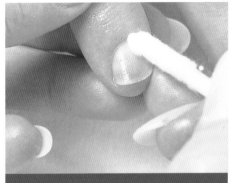

6 Firmly, but gently, push back the cuticle using the cotton bud.

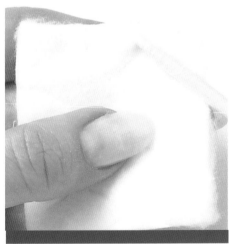

5 Make a cotton bud by wrapping an orange stick in some absorbent cotton.

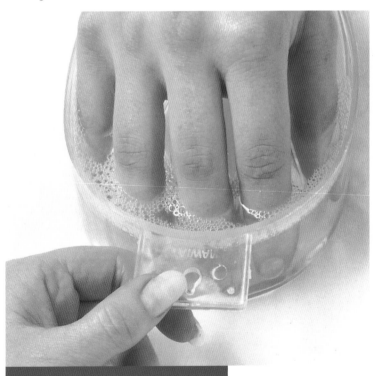

7 Repeat for the other fingers, then rinse off the oil in a bowl of water. Here we are using a professional manicurist's bowl, but any bowl or container is suitable.

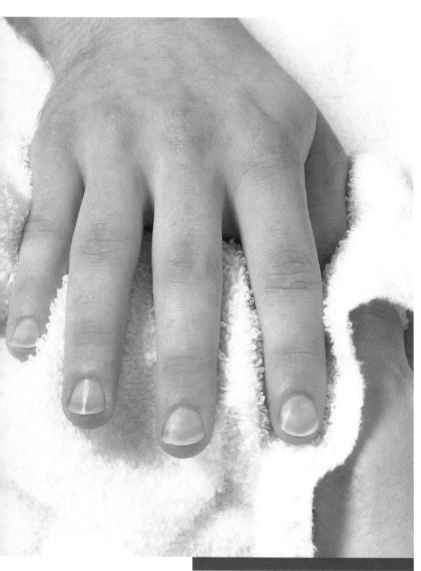

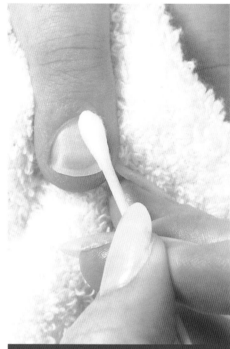

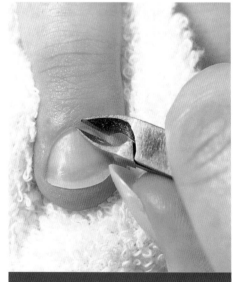

9 Use the cotton pad to push the cuticle back once more.

8 Pat the fingers dry with a soft towel.

26

10 You may see rough edges on the cuticle. You can remove these using clippers, but be careful not to cut too much. It may be better to get this done professionally if you have very ragged cuticles.

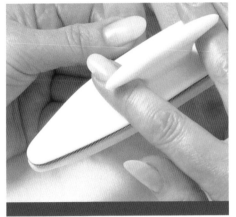

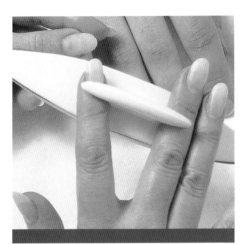

13 Repeat on the other hand, and give the nails a final buffing for a really clean and healthy shine.

Once you are used to this procedure, it will take only a few minutes to complete, and the difference will be remarkable!

11 A relaxing hand massage, as detailed on page 28, should follow. Now buff the nails. Here we are using a professional buffing pad. They are cheap to buy, and achieve a very clean effect, so buying one is recommended.

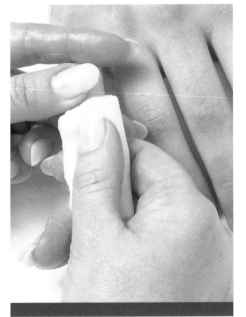

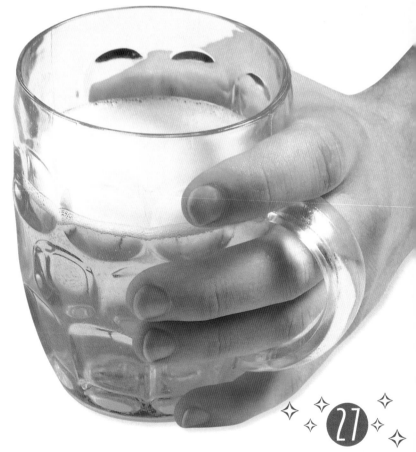

12 Now apply some nail-protecting oil with a cotton pad. Cover the whole nail area and allow to dry.

Basic Hand Massage

Massage is a very important part of a manicure. It improves the blood circulation around the nail beds, helps to keep joints supple, and eases tension in the hands and wrists, making it particularly beneficial if you use a keyboard.

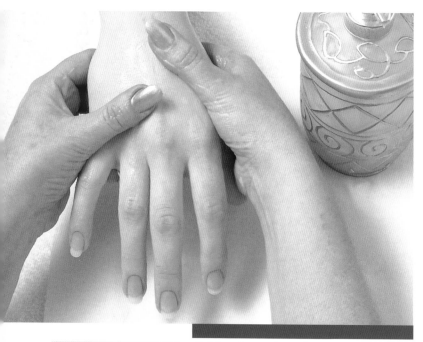

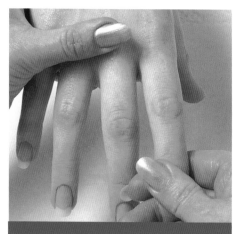

2 Taking each finger in turn, gently pull and squeeze the tip to stimulate blood flow, and release tension by pulling each finger toward you.

You Will Need

Hand cream

✧

Cotton gloves

1 After shaping the nails and treating the cuticles, a luxurious hand massage will reinvigorate stiff or tired hands. Apply a generous amount of cream to one hand, spread it evenly over each side, and massage it in using circular movements. Place your thumb and forefinger firmly, but gently, on the hand, and rotate them in a circular motion over all four fingers and thumb.

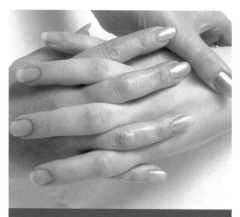

3 Ask your subject to interlock their fingers and squeeze them together, so you can massage the palms together at the same time.

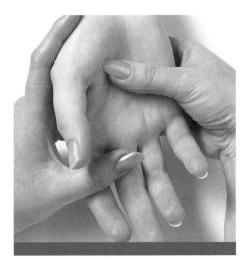

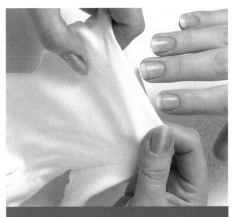

4 Holding firmly, gently rotate the hand so that the palm is facing upward, and massage it as before with both thumbs.

5 To ensure the maximum benefit from the treatment, finish off by cocooning the subject's hands in cotton gloves.

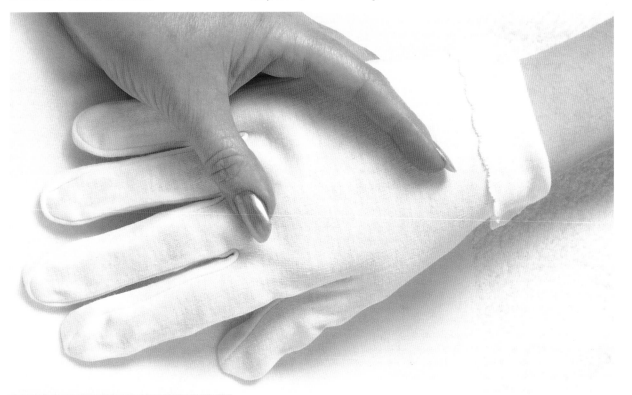

6 Keep the gloves on for at least five minutes. This antiageing strategy will intensively hydrate the hands. Now repeat the whole process on the other hand.

Pedicure

Care for your feet as well as you care for your hands – they are a vital part of your body, and deserve looking after!

You Will Need

Finest grain emery
board
✧
Cuticle gel spray (or
cuticle cream)
✧
Clippers
✧
Hard-skin
remover/pumice
stone

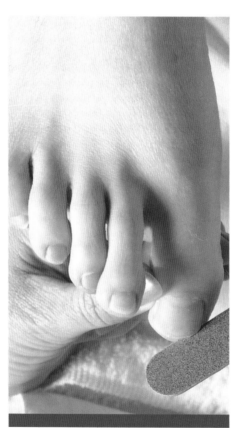

1 After soaking your feet to soften the nails, file each nail across the top. Never use a sawing motion – always file in one direction only. Never file down the sides of your nails, as this could lead to ingrowing toenails.

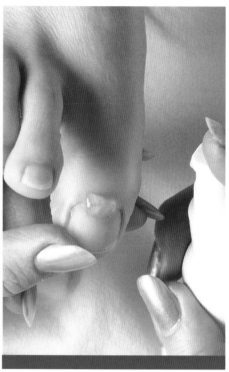

2 Apply a cuticle cream or gel (shown here in spray form) to each cuticle, and massage it in gently.

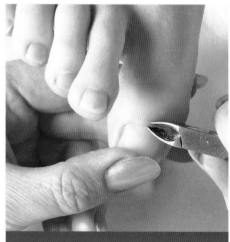

3 If you have ragged cuticles, you can trim them with clippers. However, it may be best to leave this to a professional if your cuticles are very overgrown.

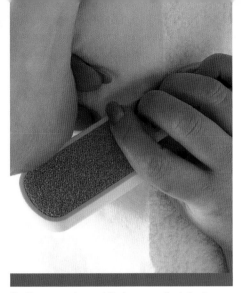

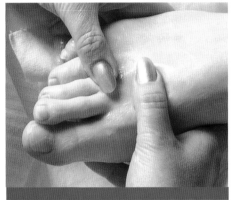

4 Once you have tidied your nails, it is time to treat the rest of your foot. The heel is one of the prime areas for building up hard skin. Buff the heel gently with an abrading tool. This could be a special hard-skin remover, a pumice stone, or loofa.

5 Now massage your feet, beginning by gently kneading across the top of your foot and across the toes.

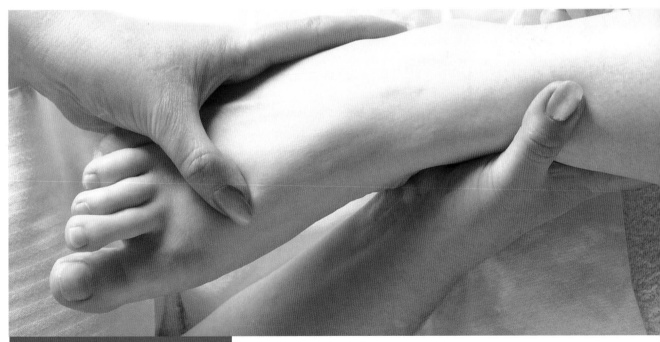

6 Finish your foot massage by working the whole foot, using your thumbs and fingers to relax and soothe. Once you have finished your pedicure, you can use any of the techniques shown in the following projects to decorate and adorn your feet.

31

Perfect French Polish

Various techniques can be used to create a perfect French polish, and you can buy special kits that guide you through the process step by step. Remember that it is important to achieve a straight "smile line" (this is the line separating the white tip from the main part of your nail). If you have a very steady hand, you will find this easy to do freehand, but if you are not confident, follow the French-tip guide to be on the safe side.

You Will Need

Base coat
✧
Pale-colored nail enamel
✧
French-tip guide tape
✧
White nail enamel
✧
Quick-drying clear topcoat

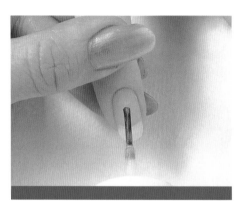

1 Apply a base coat to your nails, followed by two coats of pale-colored enamel.

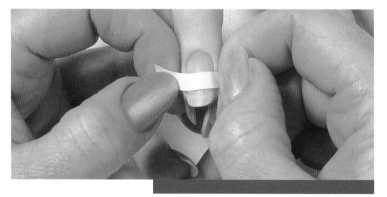

2 Having made sure that your enamel is totally dry, place the French-tip guide tape under the smile lines of the nails on either your left or right hand (it is best to work on one hand at a time).

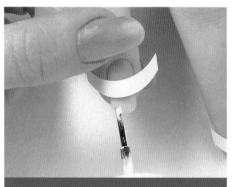

3 Carefully apply a coat of white enamel, taking it from one side of the free edge to the other. Wait for about ten minutes to allow the first coat to dry before applying a second using the same method.

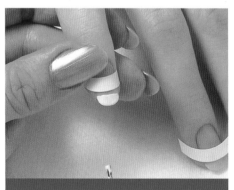

4 Follow the same procedure on your other hand (until you become more confident this will usually take a little longer).

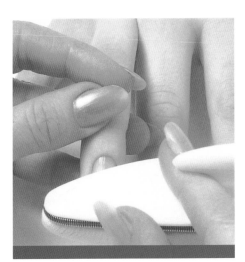

5 Now buff the whole of each nail, for a smooth finish.

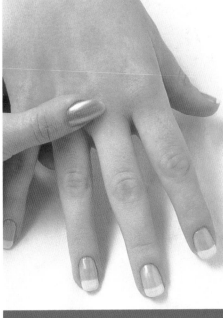

7 Your finished nails will have a truly professional look.

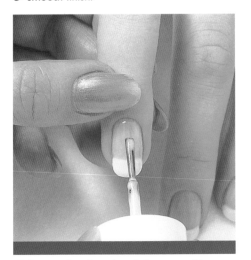

6 For a softer French polish, you could now apply pale enamel to your entire nail. If you do this, however, make sure that the white enamel is completely dry, otherwise you will smudge or drag it.

Professional tip:
I recommend that you invest in a quick-drying topcoat that contains anti-U.V. ingredients and is designed to prevent your French polish from discoloring, see index for reference.

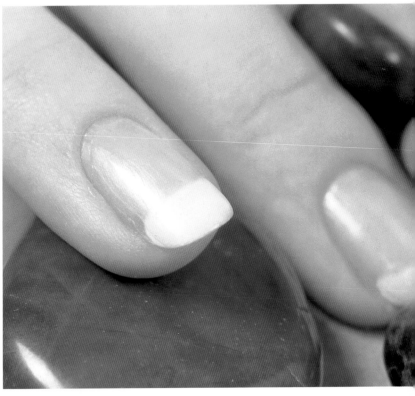

Nail Style

In the Mood

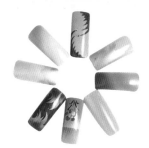

Mood-reactive enamels are a fun way to change the appearance of your nails. Watch the color darken as it reacts to the cold – or lighten as your hands warm up. Rhinestones or jewels can be added for extra effect. See the next chapter for full details on applying nail jewels.

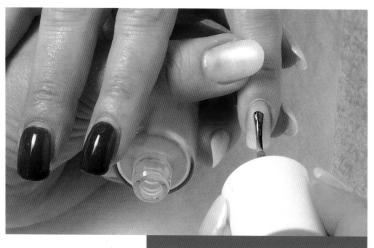

You Will Need

Base coat

⬦

Mood-tone nail enamel (color optional)

⬦

Quick-drying clear topcoat

1 Apply a base coat to each of your nails and allow it to dry thoroughly

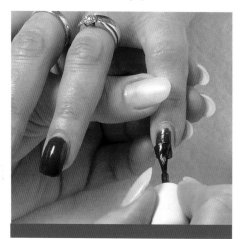

2 Apply two or three coats of your chosen mood-tone enamel.

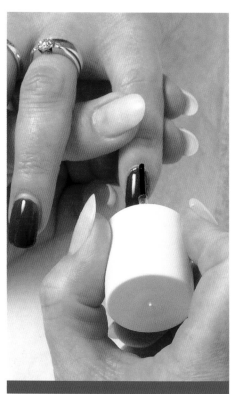

3 Having allowed the mood-tone enamel to dry completely, apply a topcoat.

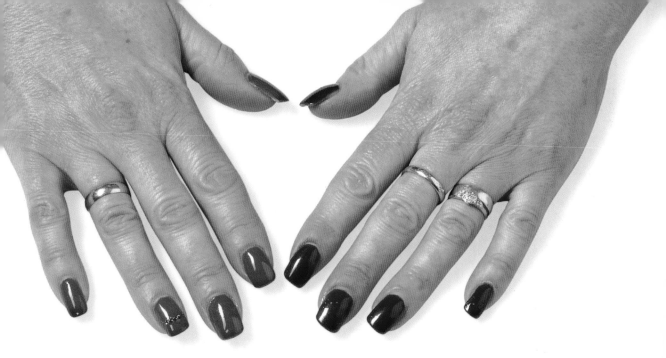

This is a stunning effect you can vary at will. The rhinestones make a stunning contrast to the varying nail color.

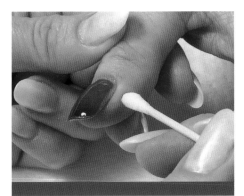

4 Using a cotton bud or pad, remove any enamel drips or marks from your fingers.

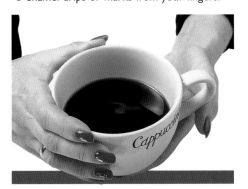

5 Here you can see the nails lighten in color as the temperature rises.

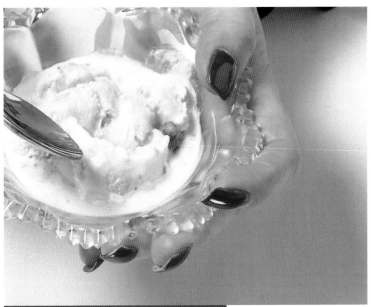

6 Coming into contact with something cold makes the color darken.

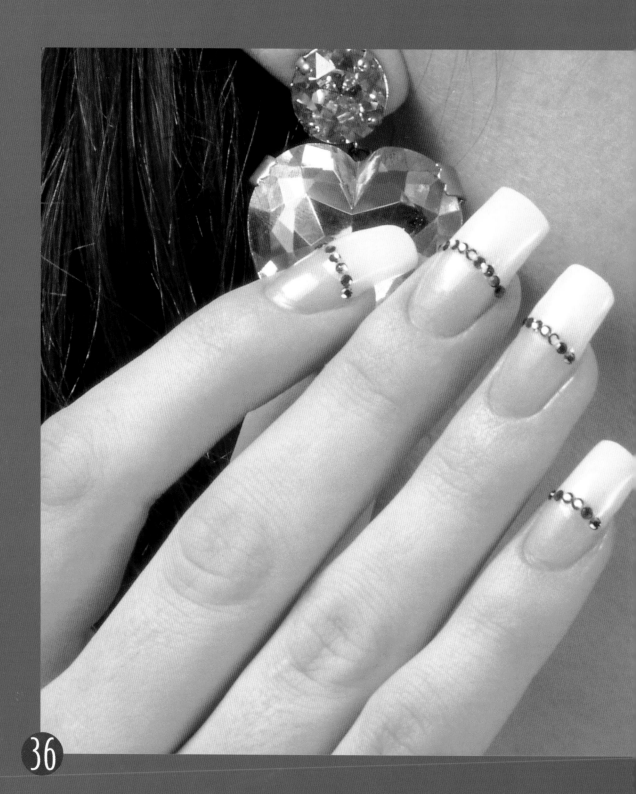

Enamel-secure Designs

Nail-art accessories can be used to create all manner of different looks. You can complement your nails with rhinestones, foil leaves, charms, studs, pearls, flat stones, and art tapes – or anything you wish!

These nail decorations are referred to as "enamel-secure," as they are applied to tacky nail enamel which acts as a bonding agent to hold the accessories securely.

Start by laying the decorations either on a sheet of nongreasy paper or in a shallow container, flat side down. Use the moistened end of an orange stick to lift and position decorations. Tweezers are useful for positioning larger decorations.

Stick-on nail art, primarily self-adhesive art tapes, are available in a number of colors, sizes, and styles, and their adhesive backing can easily be removed.

Art tapes are also easily combined with enamel-secure nail art, so you can use your imagination to create some wild and wonderful patterns and designs.

The art tapes are self-adhesive, so your nail enamel does not need to be tacky. If you wish to add some other accessories, such as rhinestones, dab on a few spots of clear topcoat to act as a bonding agent.

Once you have positioned the design on your nail, seal it in place with a clear topcoat. Make sure that you apply both base and topcoats smoothly and evenly, taking great care not to smudge your design.

Bindi Magic

This look can be particularly startling with dark enamels. Although bindi nail-art designs are sold in a variety of colors and qualities, it is best to pay a little more in order to obtain a professional finish.

You Will Need

Base coat
✧
Black nail enamel
✧
Quick-drying
clear topcoat
✧
Orange stick
✧
Container of water
✧
Bindi nail-art designs

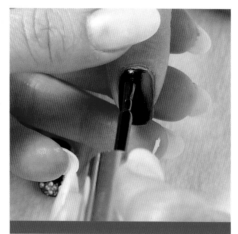

1 Apply the base coat and allow it to dry. Then apply two coats of black nail enamel. Remember not to allow the second coat to dry completely.

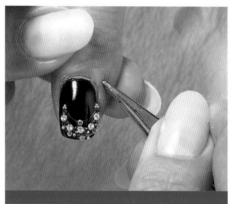

3 Dampen the end of the orange stick in the container of water and use the damp tip to pick up the bindi. While the nail enamel is still wet, position the bindi designs as you require.

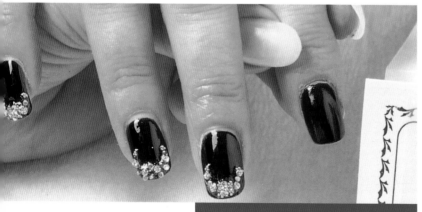

2 Select the bindi jewelry to fit the size and shape of your nail.

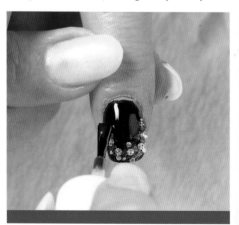

4 Seal with a topcoat. Repeat on as many other nails as you wish.

You Will Need

Base coat

✦

Black or dark-blue
nail enamel

✦

Neon strips of
nail-art tape

✦

Tweezers

✦

Orange stick

✦

Small pair of scissors

✦

Quick-drying clear
topcoat

Runway

This is a quick nail-art design that is available in a range of
colors and looks especially effective with dark enamels.

1 Apply the base coat to all of your nails and apply two
coats of black or dark-blue nail enamel.

2 When your nails are almost completely dry, use tweezers
to place one strip of tape slightly to the left of center
on your nail, from the cuticle to the tip.

3 Secure the tape firmly in place with the
orange stick . Cut the excess tape at the free edge.

4 Now place a second strip slightly to the right of center
on your nail and secure and trim as before.

5 Apply the quick-drying topcoat and allow
it to dry thoroughly.

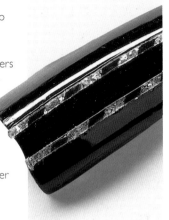

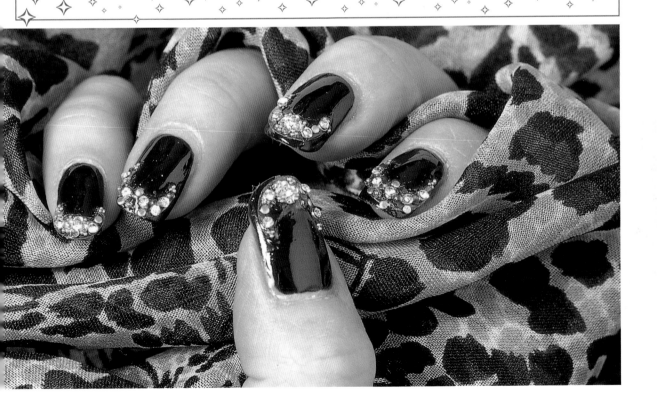

Anchors Away

You Will Need

Base coat

✧

Red nail enamel

✧

Quick-drying
clear topcoat

✧

Gold charms

✧

Orange stick

✧

Container of water

✧

Tweezers

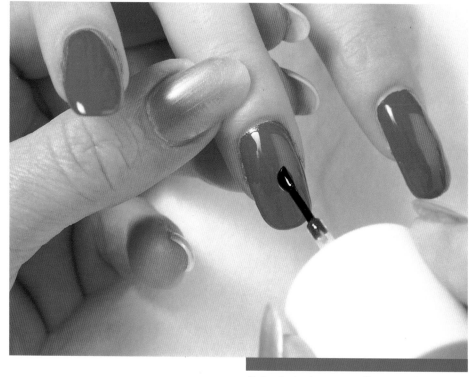

1 Apply the base coat, allow it to dry, and add two coats of red nail enamel.

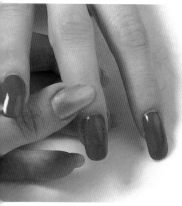

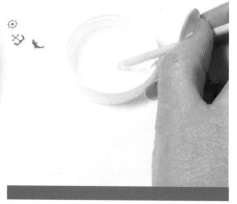

2 While the polish is tacky, you can apply the jewels by using a dampened orange stick, as in the previous project.

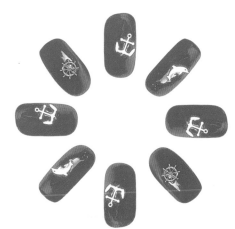

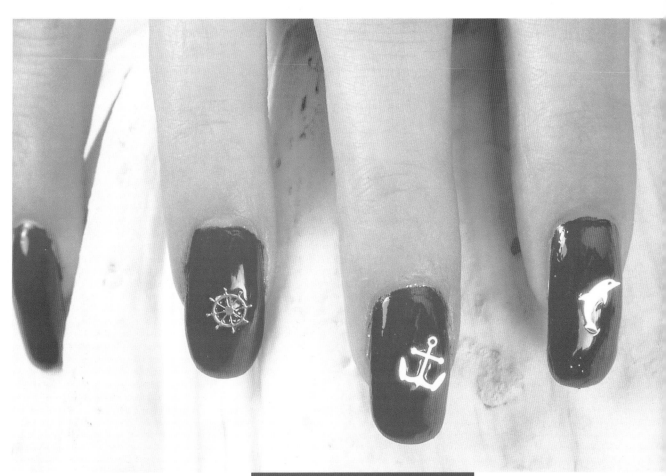

4 Once you are happy with the layout of your charms, apply the topcoat. This is a design that looks stunning on one nail, with the others finished in plain enamel. However, you can apply charms to as many nails as you wish.

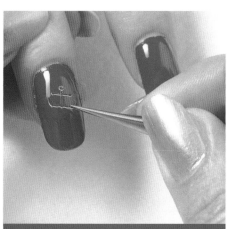

3 Alternatively, you can use tweezers to pick up and position the charms.

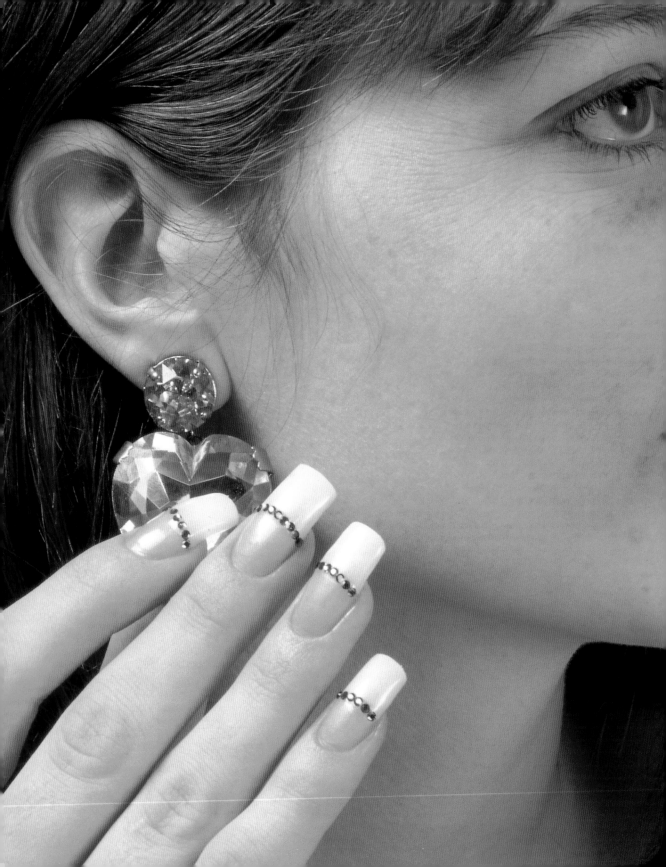

Glittering Prize

This stylish design borrows from the classic French polish to create an elegant and understated finish – perfect for glamorous occasions.

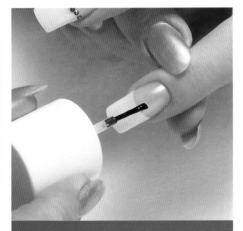

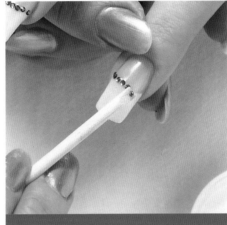

You Will Need

Clear base coat
✧
Quick-drying
clear topcoat
✧
Green rhinestones
✧
Orange stick
✧
Container of water

1 Apply the base coat, and once this has dried, apply the topcoat. Do not allow to dry completely.

3 Continue placing the rhinestones until they form a glittering band across the whole smile line.

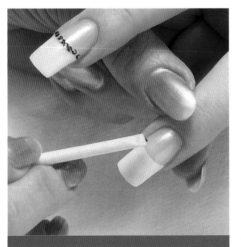

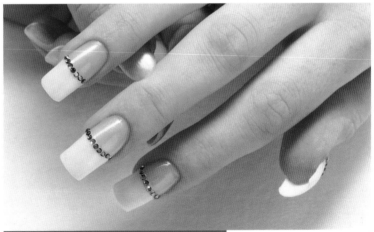

2 Using the dampened tip of the orange stick, apply the first rhinestone, beginning at the edge of your smile line.

4 This is a very sophisticated look, so will look best if you apply the design to all of your nails, rather than just one.

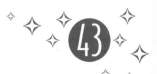

Casino Lady

This is a variation on the previous project, and uses colored enamel and a diagonal line of rhinestones for a glitzy look.

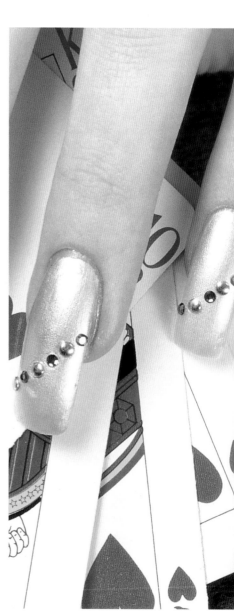

You Will Need

Clear base coat

✧

Silver nail enamel

✧

Quick-drying clear topcoat

✧

Green rhinestones

✧

Orange stick

✧

Container of water

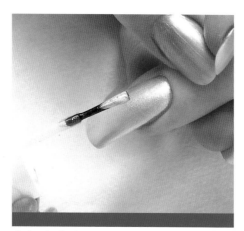

1 Apply the base coat, allow it to dry, and apply two coats of silver nail enamel.

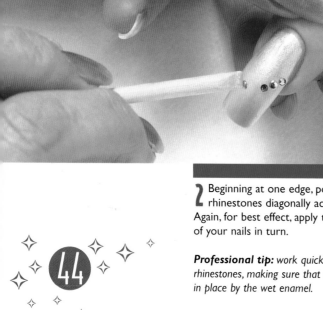

2 Beginning at one edge, position the rhinestones diagonally across your nail. Again, for best effect, apply the design to each of your nails in turn.

Professional tip: *work quickly when positioning rhinestones, making sure that each is securely held in place by the wet enamel.*

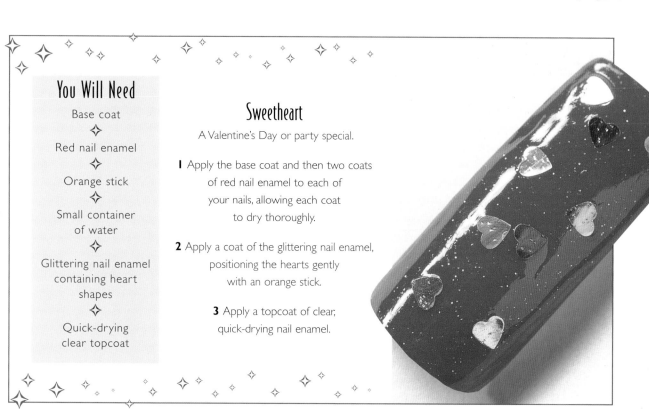

You Will Need

Base coat

✧

Red nail enamel

✧

Orange stick

✧

Small container
of water

✧

Glittering nail enamel
containing heart
shapes

✧

Quick-drying
clear topcoat

Sweetheart

A Valentine's Day or party special.

1 Apply the base coat and then two coats
of red nail enamel to each of
your nails, allowing each coat
to dry thoroughly.

2 Apply a coat of the glittering nail enamel,
positioning the hearts gently
with an orange stick.

3 Apply a topcoat of clear,
quick-drying nail enamel.

You Will Need

Base coat

✧

Your own choice
of colored
nail enamel

✧

Tweezers

✧

Charms

✧

Quick-drying
clear topcoat

Kiss Me Quick

For a more subtle approach, try this on one
nail only.

1 Apply a base coat and two coats
of colored nail enamel.

2 While the enamel is still wet,
secure each charm in turn.
Allow the nail enamel to dry.

3 Seal in the charms with quick-drying
topcoat. Apply two coats, allowing the first
to dry before applying the second.

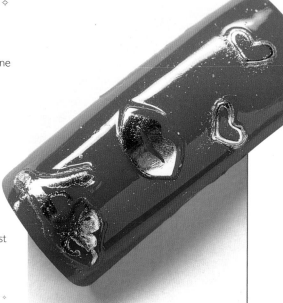

Lace With a Twist

You can create your own enamel-secure design by using lace for a delicate, textured effect. Contrast the ultrafeminine, lacy look with some leather accessories for some rock-chick glamor!

You Will Need

Base coat

✧

Candy-pink
nail enamel

✧

Small pair
of scissors

✧

Piece of lace

✧

Orange stick

✧

Quick-drying clear
topcoat

✧

Rhinestones or
pearls (optional)

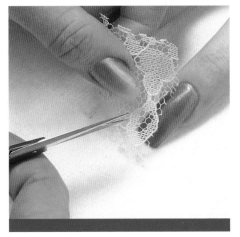

1 Cut and shape the lace so that it matches the shape and size of your nails.

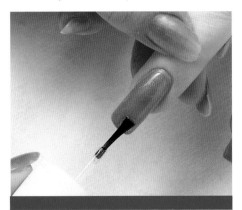

2 Apply the base coat to each nail, followed by two coats of candy-pink nail enamel. When this has dried, apply a clear topcoat.

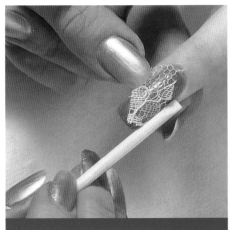

3 Place the lace over the slightly tacky surface of the nail. Using an orange stick, maneuver it into place, taking care not to stain the lace. Carefully cut any frayed edges.

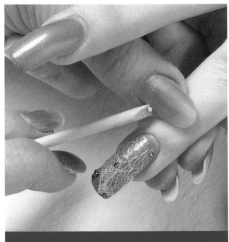

4 Add one or more rhinestones to complete the effect.

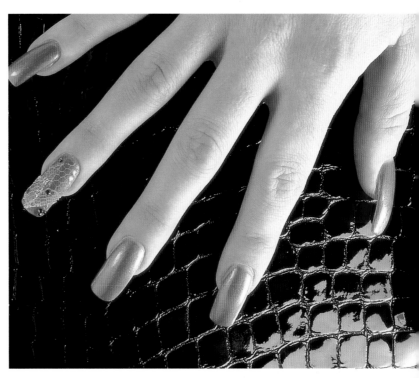

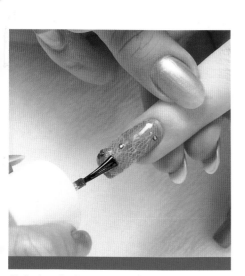

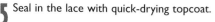

5 Seal in the lace with quick-drying topcoat.

You Will Need

Base coat

✧

White nail enamel

✧

Quick-drying
clear topcoat

✧

Tweezers

✧

Stick-on eyes

Here's Looking at You, Kid

An "eye-catching," fun design!

1 Apply base coat followed by two coats of white nail enamel.

2 Position the stick-on eyes – as many, and wherever you wish.

3 As the eyes stand proud of the nails, it is not practical to add a final topcoat.

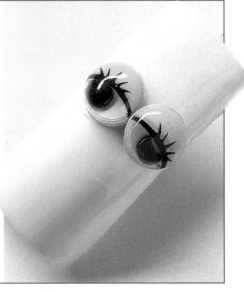

47

Starlight Express

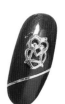

A combination of rhinestones and arty tape makes this a stunning party design. Charms can be added if required. You can continue the design on every nail, but you may find it more effective to leave some nails plain.

You Will Need

Base coat
✧
Electric-blue
nail enamel
✧
Silver nail-art tape
✧
Small pair
of scissors
✧
Orange stick
✧
Container of water
✧
4 rhinestones per
nail
✧
Quick-drying
clear topcoat

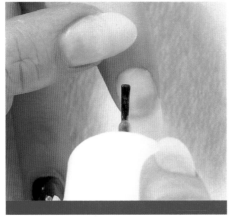

1 Apply the base coat to all of your nails. Allow this to dry.

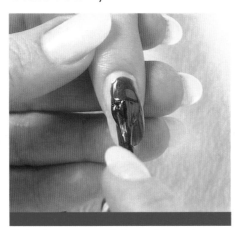

2 Apply two coats of electric-blue nail enamel and allow to dry thoroughly.

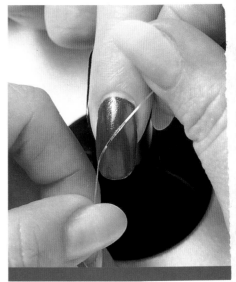

3 Cut a length of silver nail-art tape to the correct length. Place it on the nail so that it runs diagonally from corner to corner.

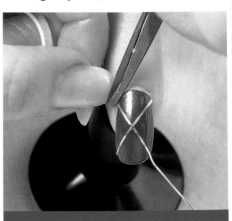

4 Now place another length of tape on the nail so that it runs from the opposite corner to corner and crosses the first tape.

You Will Need

Base coat

✧

Your own choice of
colored
nail enamel

✧

Orange stick

✧

Small container
of water

✧

Tiny rhinestones
(7 per nail)

✧

Quick-drying
clear topcoat

Rhinestone Daisy

This rhinestone flower is particularly effective for
making one nail stand out.

1 Apply a base coat, followed by two coats of
colored nail enamel.

2 Position the first rhinestone in
the center of your nail.

3 Next, place one rhinestone above the central
rhinestone and one below, making sure that they
are evenly spaced.

4 Using the same method, place the remaining
four rhinestones so that they complete the circle.

5 Finish by applying a topcoat of clear nail enamel.

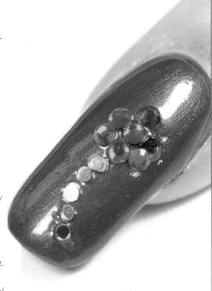

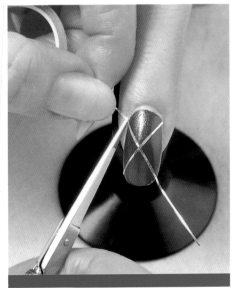

5 Trim the ends of the tape so it fits the
shape of your nail.

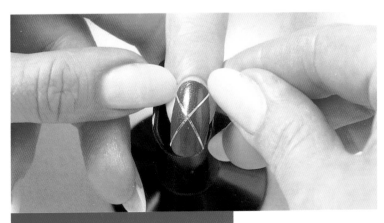

6 Loose tape may catch on clothes and tear,
so make sure you fix the ends of the tape
securely into the enamel, following the shape
of your nail.

49

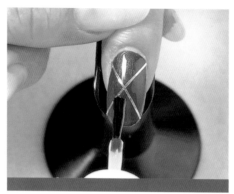

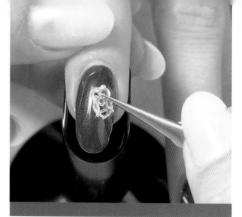

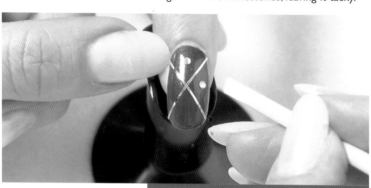

9 You can add a silver charm to one or more of your nails as a finishing touch. Here we have added a tiny owl.

7 Apply one coat of topcoat as a bonding agent for the rhinestones, leaving it tacky.

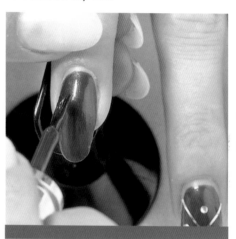

8 Now place four rhinestones on each nail, positioning them so that they are centered within the spaces between the tapes.

10 Seal with a topcoat and allow this to dry thoroughly.

50

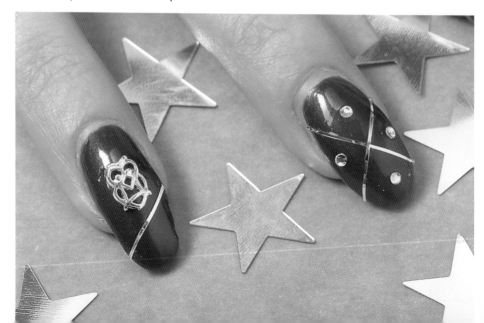

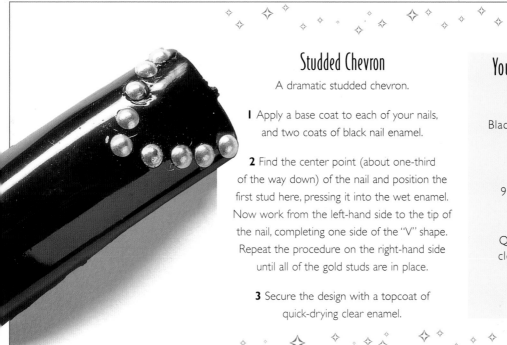

Studded Chevron

A dramatic studded chevron.

1 Apply a base coat to each of your nails, and two coats of black nail enamel.

2 Find the center point (about one-third of the way down) of the nail and position the first stud here, pressing it into the wet enamel. Now work from the left-hand side to the tip of the nail, completing one side of the "V" shape. Repeat the procedure on the right-hand side until all of the gold studs are in place.

3 Secure the design with a topcoat of quick-drying clear enamel.

You Will Need

Base coat

✧

Black nail enamel

✧

Tweezers

✧

9 gold studs per nail

✧

Quick-drying clear topcoat

You Will Need

Base coat

✧

Magenta nail enamel

✧

3 strips of holographic nail-art tape per nail (cut to nail length)

✧

Small pair of scissors

✧

Orange stick

✧

Quick-drying clear topcoat

Tram Lines

See how the holographic tape catches the light.

1 Apply the base coat to all of your nails and then apply two coats of magenta nail enamel.

2 Apply the holographic tape diagonally across the nail (from bottom left to top right). Use an orange stick to press it down carefully.

3 Using the second length of tape, repeat the procedure from bottom right to top left.

4 Finally, position the last piece of tape up the center of the nail. Cut off any excess tape when you reach the tip of the nail.

5 Secure the design with a topcoat of quick-drying clear nail enamel.

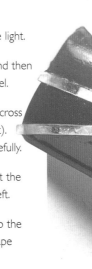

Emerald Isle

This is a truly stunning combination of techniques! A Gaelic motif has been stenciled so that it runs up the side of the foot to the ankle.

The toenails have been painted with emerald-green and gold nail enamel. The rhinestones on the feet and the gold studs have been taken diagonally across, from corner to corner.

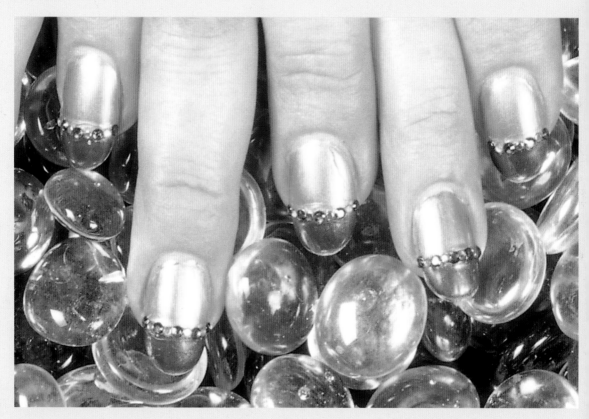

Although the French-manicure design on the hands was created with the same colors, the rhinestones were placed across the smile line, running from one edge of the nail to the other.

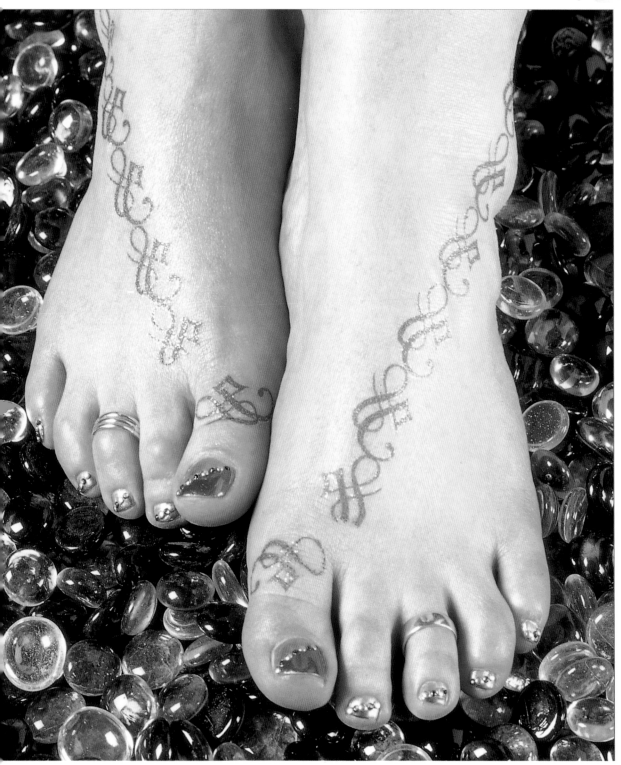

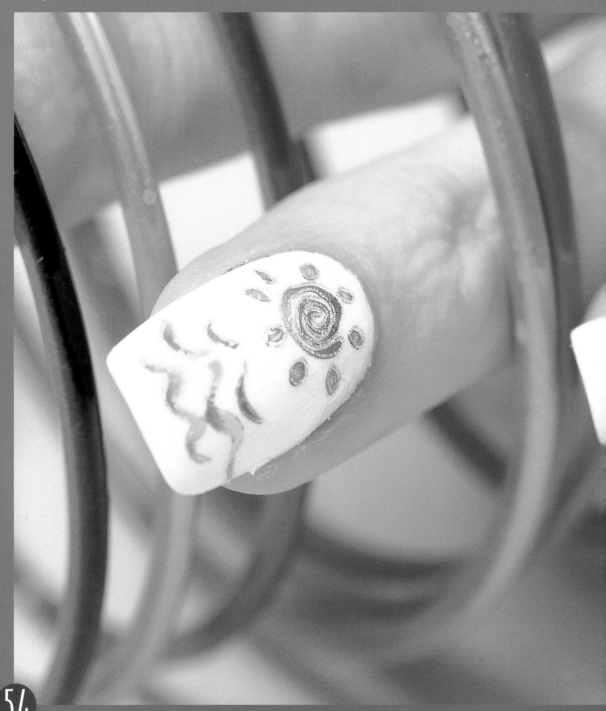

Transfers and Decals

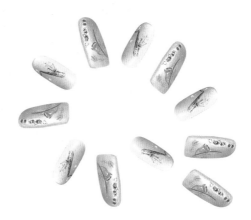

A nail-art transfer, also known as a decal, is usually formatted on a background of white gloss paper, which, when it comes into contact with water, releases the picture film onto the nail surface. Depending on the type of nail art and design, you can use these films on either an unpainted nail or an enameled one. They are easily removed with acetone-free nail-enamel remover.

If you are feeling rather more adventurous, you could combine transfers with other forms of nail art, such as rhinestones and foil tapes, to create an individual look.

There are a number of ways of removing a decal from its backing sheet. You can soak the decal face down in a small container of water, until the decal slides easily off the backing sheet. However, some decals are of poor quality, and soaking them may make

them disintegrate. My professional tip is to use a few drops of water and a cotton bud to dampen the back of the decal. It can take about 30 seconds for the paper to absorb the water and release the transfer. You may sometimes have to dampen the decal more than once.

Both methods are variously employed in the following projects. It is up to you which method you choose.

Dancing Butterflies

A delicate effect that is ideal for a romantic summer day – it is also an especially pretty style for a bride.

You Will Need

Base coat

❖

Pale nail enamel

❖

Small pair of scissors

❖

Decals

❖

Bowl of water

❖

Cotton bud

❖

Tweezers

❖

Quick-drying clear topcoat

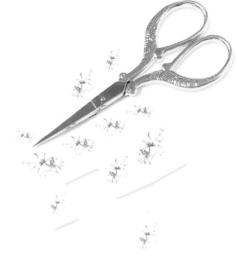

1 First select and cut out your decal, making sure it will fit the size and shape of your nail. Size each nail separately.

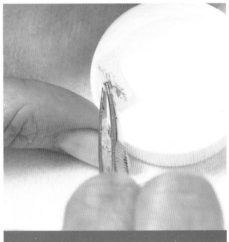

3 Now apply two coats of pale nail enamel, again allowing each coat to dry thoroughly.

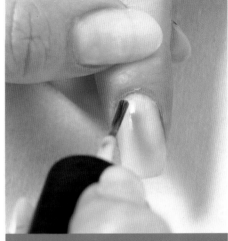

4 Place the decal face down in a container of water. Use tweezers to hold the edge.

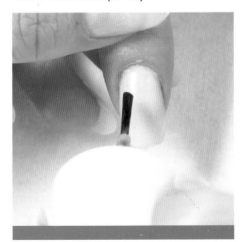

2 Apply a base coat, allowing it to dry completely.

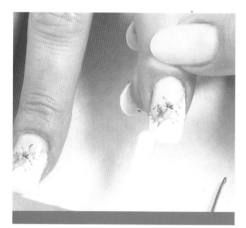

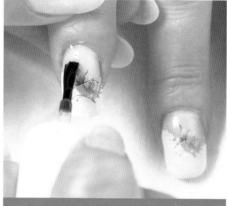

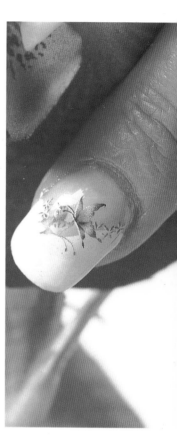

5 Carefully pick up your backing sheet with the tweezers and turn it over so that you can see the design. Using a slightly dampened cotton bud, line up the decal with your polished nail. Slide the decal off the backing sheet and position with the cotton bud.

6 When you are happy with the position of the design, apply the quick-drying topcoat. It is vital that you do not drag the brush over your design.

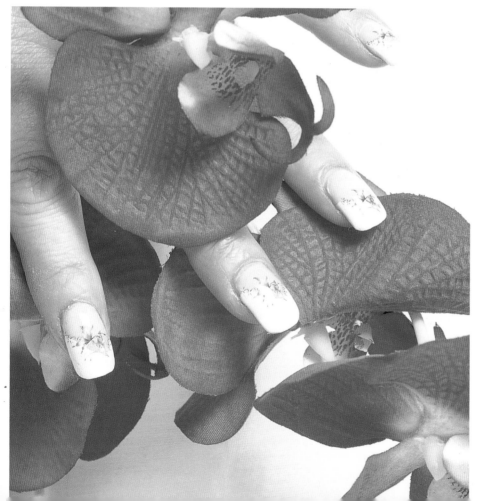

57

The Big Blue

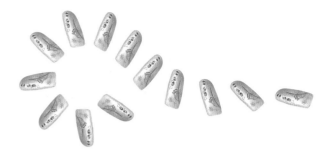

Using complementary nail-enamel colours, you can achieve your own fantasy wonderland or seascape. For this design we have used tiny sections of decals, cutting them into individual shapes to create our own "big blue."

You Will Need

Base coat

✧

Ocean-blue
nail enamel

✧

Small pair of scissors

✧

Decals

✧

Bowl of water

✧

Cotton bud

✧

Tweezers

✧

Quick-drying
clear topcoat

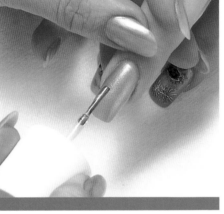
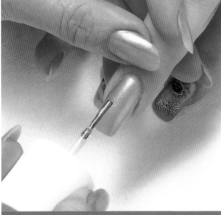

1 Apply the base coat to all of your nails, followed by two coats of ocean-blue nail enamel. Allow each coat to dry thoroughly.

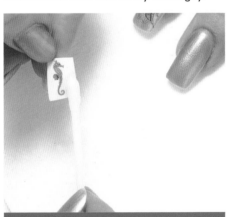

2 Select and cut out the first decal. This will form the basis of your seascape.

3 To build up your fantasy scene, choose other decals whose size and pattern complement your first choice.

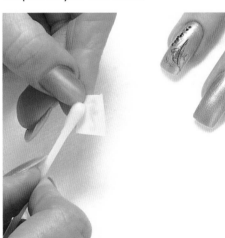

4 Holding the decal with the tweezers, use a damp cotton bud to moisten the back of the first decal.

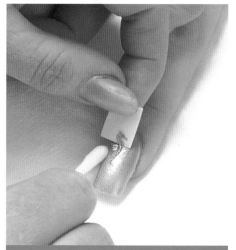

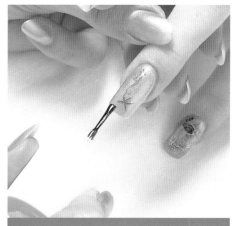

5 Place the first decal onto your nail, ensuring that it does not wrinkle.

7 Seal your design with a quick-drying topcoat, taking care not to drag the brush over your nail art.

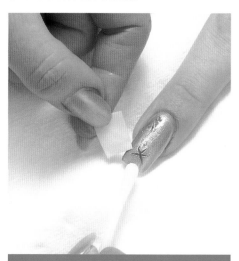

6 Now position the remaining decals to create a beautiful undersea scene.

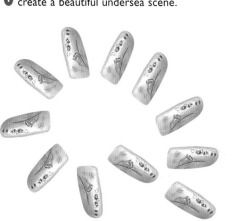

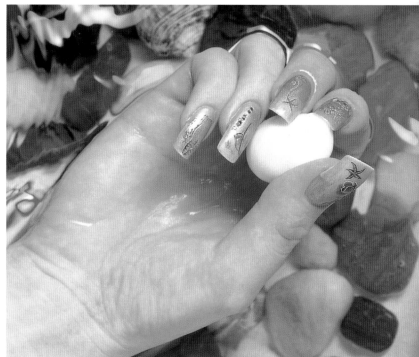

59

Hollywood Glitz

Bring some award-night glamor to your nails with these fun golden decals.

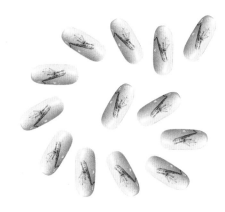

You Will Need

Base coat

✧

White nail enamel

✧

Small pair of scissors

✧

Decals

✧

Bowl of water

✧

Cotton bud

✧

Tweezers

✧

Quick-drying clear topcoat

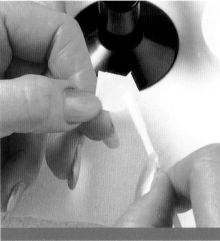

1 Apply the base coat, followed by two coats of white nail enamel, allowing each coat to dry thoroughly. Choose your decals and wet the first using a cotton bud.

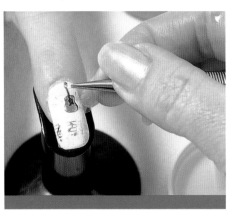

2 Position the decal using tweezers, making sure that the transfer does not wrinkle.

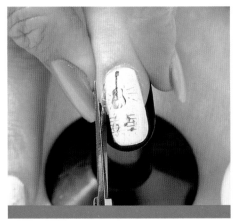

3 Place the remaining decals on your nail with the tweezers. Add as many as you like – the effect you want is over-the-top glamor!

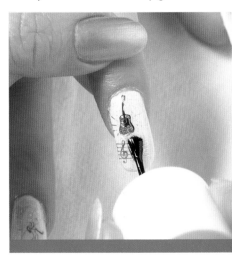

4 Seal your design with a quick-drying topcoat, taking care not to drag the brush over your nail art.

Tiptoe Through the Tulips

A pretty, feminine design that will look effective whether placed either on one nail or on all of them

You Will Need

Base coat	Bowl of water
Pale nail enamel	Tweezers
Glitter enamel (optional)	Cotton bud
Small pair of scissors	Container of water
Transfers	Quick-drying clear topcoat

1 Apply the base coat to all of your nails, followed by two coats of pale nail enamel, allowing each coat to dry thoroughly.

2 Select and cut out your decals. Dampen the first with a cotton bud and use the tweezers to position it at the bottom of your nail, in the center.

3 Place a second tulip to the right and a third tulip to the left of the first.

4 Make sure that all of the transfers are wrinkle-free by smoothing them with a moist cotton bud.

5 Apply two coats of quick-drying topcoat, followed by a coat of glitter enamel if required.

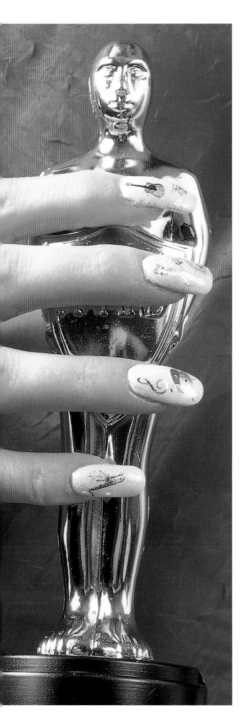

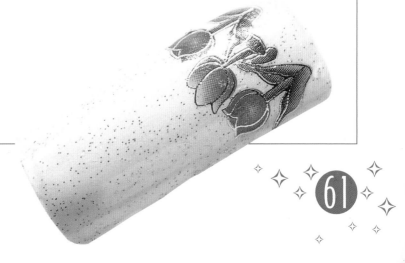

Professional tip: *you will see in this project that we are using a nail stand. These are cheap to buy and make it easier to hold the nail steady when applying decals or other nail accessories.*

Glittering Roses

Whole-nail decals are a quick and effective way to achieve glamorous nails. They come in a variety of styles, and can be matched to your favorite accessories for added effect.

You Will Need

Base coat

✧

Green nail enamel

✧

Small pair of scissors

✧

Decals

✧

Bowl of water

✧

Cotton bud

✧

Tweezers

✧

Quick-drying clear topcoat

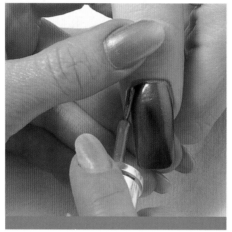

1 Apply the base coat, followed by two coats of green nail enamel, allowing each coat to dry thoroughly before continuing.

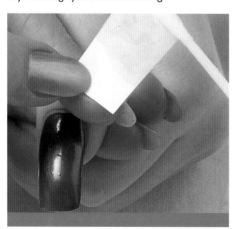

2 Choose a decal that complements the color of your polish. Wet the back of the decal with a damp cotton bud.

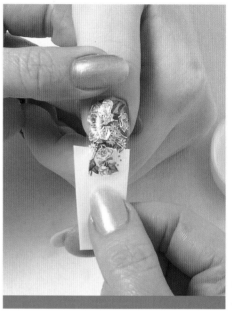

3 Begin removing the decal from the backing paper, sliding it into position on your nail.

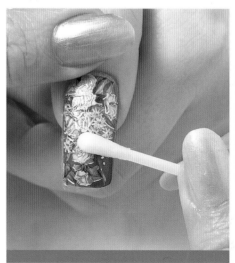

4 Secure the decal in place, using the damp cotton bud to position the decal evenly on your nail.

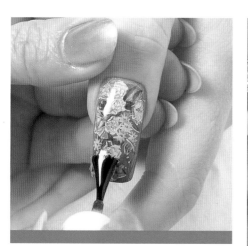

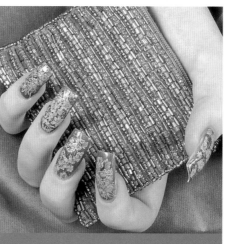

5 Seal your design with a quick-drying topcoat, taking care not to drag the brush over your nail art.

6 You can choose colors and decals that match your clothes or accessories!

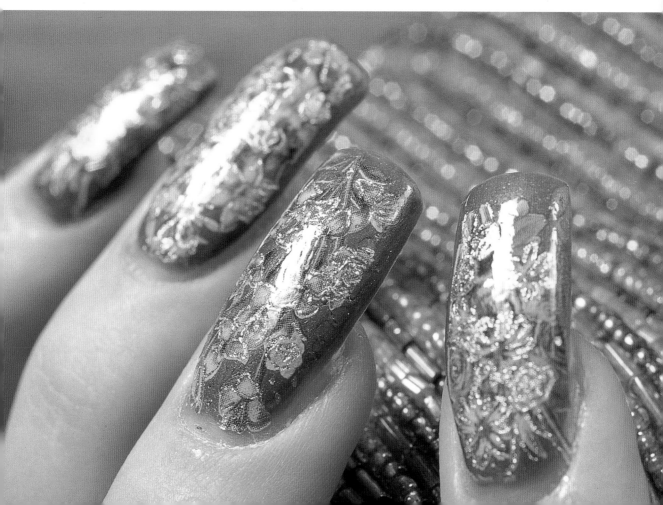

Candy Girl

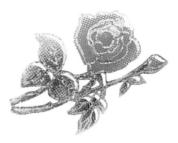

By cutting and designing your decals as if they were elements of a designer outfit, you can mix and match all sorts of colors and styles.

You Will Need

Base coat

✧

White nail enamel

✧

Small pair of scissors

✧

Decals

✧

Bowl of water

✧

Cotton bud

✧

Tweezers

✧

Quick-drying clear topcoat

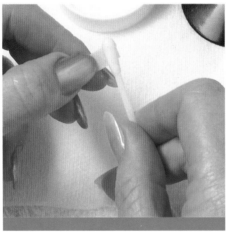

1 Apply the base coat, followed by two coats of white nail enamel, allowing each coat to dry thoroughly. Moisten the back of your first decal with a damp cotton bud.

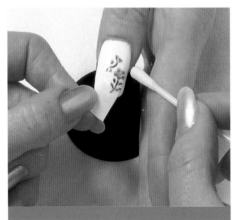

2 Slide the decal onto your nail and smooth it into place using a damp cotton bud.

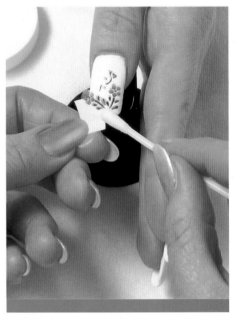

3 Apply further decals in the same way, and when you are satisfied with the design, seal with a quick-drying topcoat, taking care not to drag the brush over your nail art.

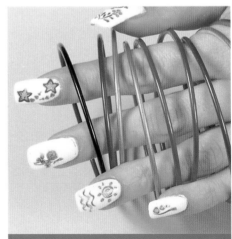

4 As with any nail art, you can choose styles and colors to match accessories.

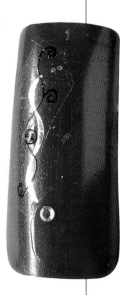

You Will Need

Base coat

Purple nail enamel

Small pair of scissors

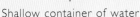

Strip of nail-art scroll tape

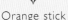

Shallow container of water

Tweezers

Rhinestones

Orange stick

Quick-drying clear topcoat

Scrolling Along

This scroll transfer comes in a special strip, so you can use as much or as little as you like.

1 Apply the base coat to all of your nails, followed by two coats of purple nail enamel.

2 Carefully cut out the scroll tape, place it face down in a little water, and allow it to soak.

3 Using tweezers, remove the scroll tape from the water and apply it down the left side of your nail. Use an orange stick to secure it, starting from the base of the nail. Cut off any excess tape once you have reached the tip of the nail.

4 Using tweezers or a dampened orange stick, pick up and position the rhinestones.

5 Secure your design with a quick-drying topcoat of clear nail enamel.

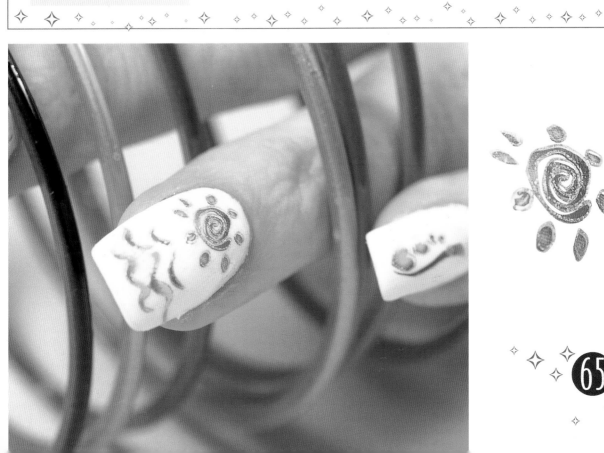

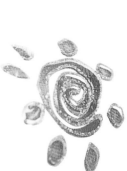

Fantasy Island

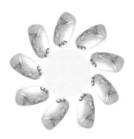

This project combines techniques from the previous chapters to create a fun scene ideal for summer nights. This design will work equally well on one nail only or as a continuous scene across each nail on your hands.

You Will Need

Base coat

✧

White nail enamel

✧

Small pair of scissors

✧

Cutout transfers
(2 per nail)

✧

Bowl of water

✧

Gold tape

✧

Orange stick

✧

Tweezers

✧

Cotton bud

✧

Blue rhinestones
(1 per nail)

✧

Iridescent rhinestones
(1 per nail)

✧

Quick-drying
clear topcoat

✧

Gold glitter enamel
(optional)

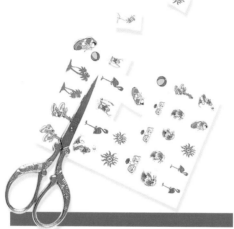

1 Carefully select the transfers you will use on each nail. For this nail we are using a palm tree.

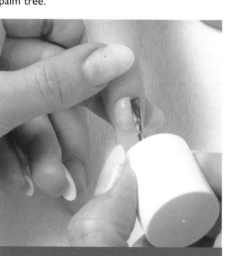

2 Apply the base coat and allow it to dry thoroughly.

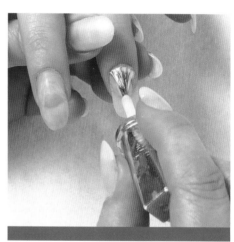

3 Now apply two coats of white nail enamel. Do not allow the second coat to dry completely – it should be slightly tacky.

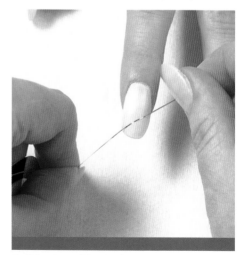

4 Take the gold tape diagonally across the lower edge of your nail, securing each edge into the wet enamel with the orange stick.

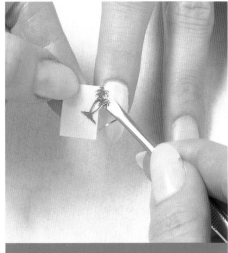

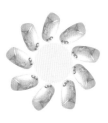

7 Pick up the transfer with the tweezers and slide it gently over your nail, making sure that the palm tree extends to the free edge and that the branches fall over the tape.

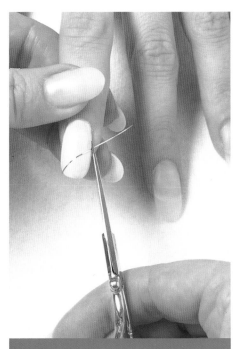

5 Trim the ends of the tape to fit your nail.

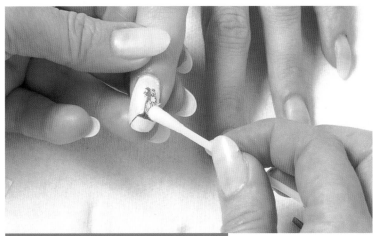

8 Use the cotton bud to smooth out any wrinkles, remembering to keep it moist only and not soaking wet.

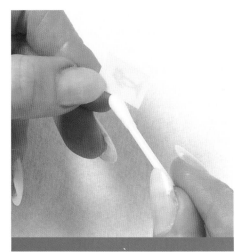

6 Dampen the end of the cotton bud and moisten the back of the palm-tree decal.

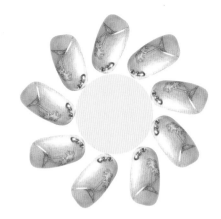

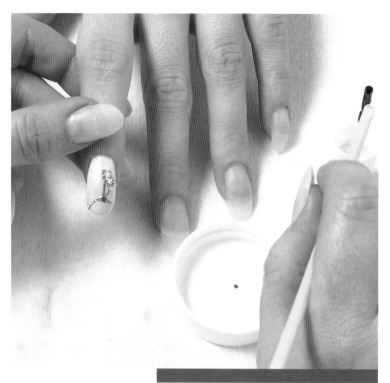

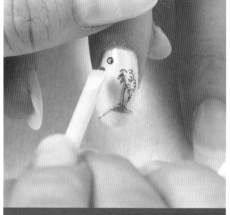

9 Dampen the tip of the orange stick and carefully pick up the first rhinestone.

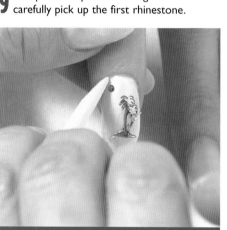

10 Place the rhinestone on the nail. If the enamel has dried, add a dab of topcoat where you want to position the rhinestone.

11 Add further rhinestones if required.

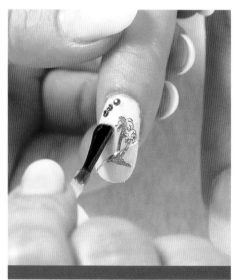

12 Seal your design with topcoat, being careful not drag the brush too heavily.

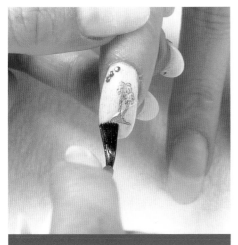

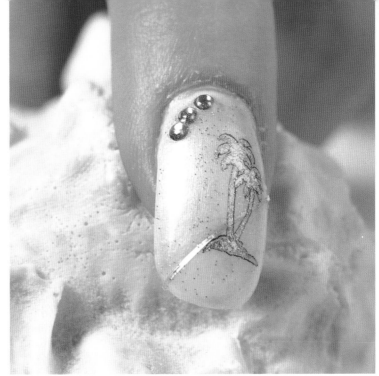

13 For that extra eye-catching effect, apply a coat of gold glitter enamel.

Queen of Hearts

Create a deck of cards across your fingers, or simply decorate one nail.

1 Apply the base coat, followed by two coats of silver nail enamel.

2 Submerge the queen of hearts transfer face down in a container of water. Using tweezers and a damp cotton bud, slide the queen of hearts decal into position at the top left-hand corner of your nail.

3 Repeat the process with the king of spades transfer, placing it on the bottom right-hand corner of your nail.

4 After you have positioned the transfers, use the moist cotton bud to pat them gently into shape, removing any excess wrinkles so that you end up with a smooth surface. Now apply the topcoat.

You Will Need

Base coat

Silver nail enamel

1 cutout transfer of the queen of hearts
and
1 cutout transfer of the king of spades

Bowl of water

Tweezers

Cotton bud

Quick-drying clear topcoat

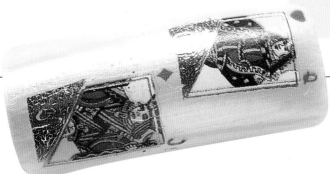

69

Snakeskin

Mood-tone enamels can be used as an attractive addition to any form of nail art. Here the green changes to yellow, complementing the snakeskin decal.

You Will need

Base coat

⬥

Pale-green mood-tone enamel

⬥

Small pair of scissors

⬥

Decals

⬥

Shallow container of water

⬥

Tweezers

⬥

Cotton bud

⬥

Quick-drying clear topcoat

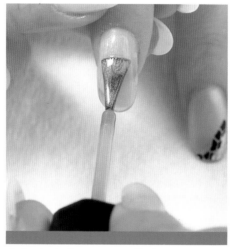

1 Apply the base coat to all of your nails. Allow this to dry thoroughly.

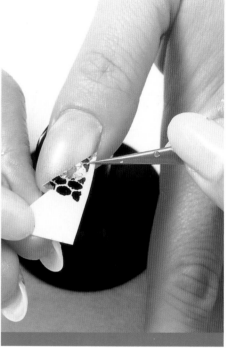

3 You will need to cut the decal to match the size of your nail exactly. Moisten the decal with a damp cotton bud and, using tweezers, gently position it across your nail.

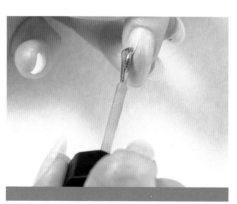

2 Now apply two coats of the mood-tone enamel and allow to dry.

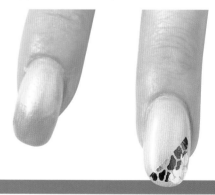

4 Shape the decal to fit your nail, using a damp cotton bud to avoid wrinkles. Then apply the quick-drying topcoat.

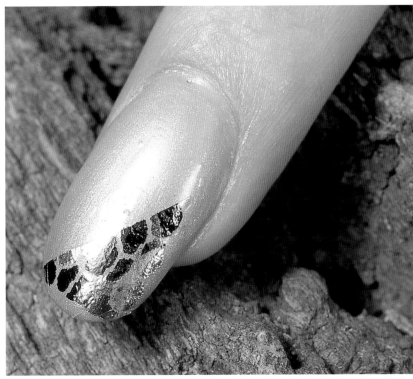

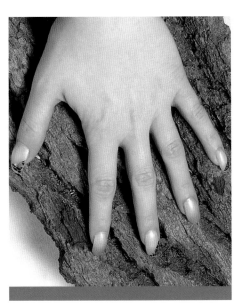

5 This is an excellent example of nail art that looks even more stunning if continued over the whole hand.

You Will Need

Base coat

✧

Pale-blue nail enamel

✧

Small pair of scissors

✧

Cutout transfers

✧

Bowl of water

✧

Tweezers

✧

Cotton bud

✧

Quick-drying clear topcoat

Surfer's Paradise

Patience is a virtue when creating this design, as you will join three different shapes together to make a single image.

I Apply the base coat to each nail, followed by two coats of enamel, allowing each coat to dry thoroughly.

2 Position one wave transfer on the bottom right-hand corner of your nail. Repeat on the left-hand side.

3 Ensure that the transfers are wrinkle-free by smoothing with a cotton bud. Secure the surfer transfer atop the wave.

4 You could also add a sun transfer or foil tape.

5 Apply two coats of top coat, making sure not to drag the brush over the design. Allow both coats to dry thoroughly.

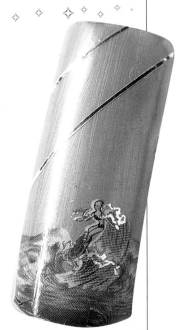

Wild Thing

A fantastic combination of techniques that will bring out the wild thing in you. It looks fabulous on feet, but can be applied as easily to hands. This design also uses transfers that can be applied to your skin.

You Will Need

Toe separators

✧

Base coat

✧

Green nail enamel

✧

Quick-drying
clear topcoat

✧

Cotton bud

✧

Cotton pads

✧

Container of water

✧

Tiger decals

✧

Barbed-wire transfer

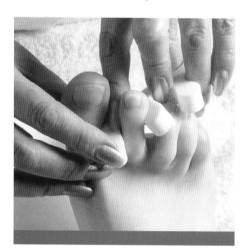

1 Position the toe separators to avoid smudging your enamel.

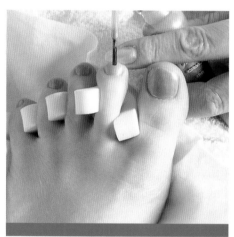

3 Apply two coats of green nail enamel and allow each to dry.

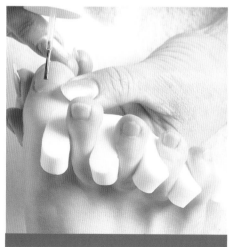

2 Apply a base coat and allow it to dry completely.

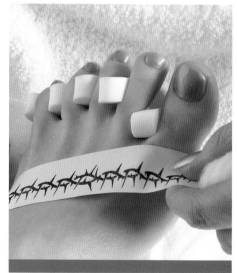

4 Choose where you want to place your barbed-wire transfer.

72

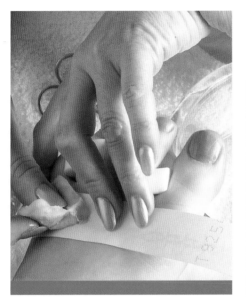

5 Carefully dampen the back of the transfer a little and place it face down in position.

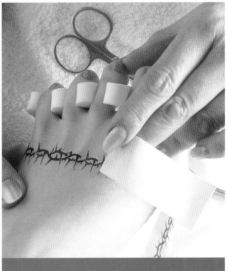

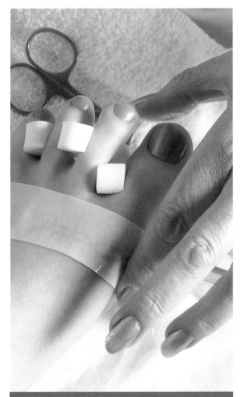

6 Using a damp cotton pad, make sure the whole back of the transfer strip is moist.

7 Gently peel away the backing strip. If part of the design still adheres to this strip, place it back down and dampen it again.

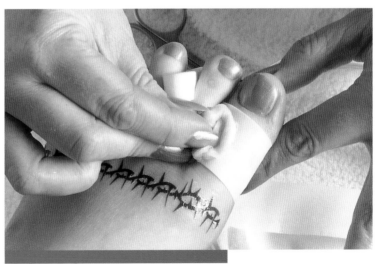

8 Now use the same technique to position a smaller strip of barbed-wire stencil across the base of your big toe.

73

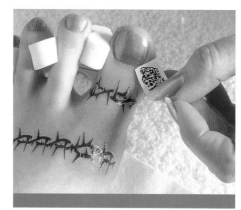

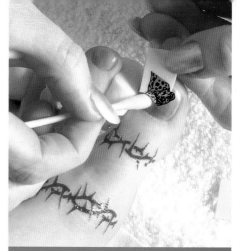

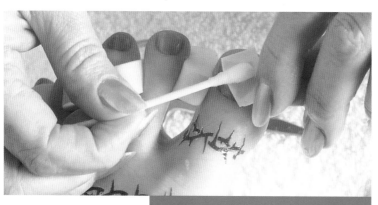

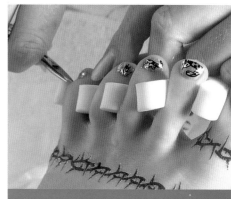

9 Next select the tiger decals to fit each of your toenails.

11 Apply the decal by sliding it into place with the cotton bud.

10 Position the first decal by dampening the back using a moist cotton bud.

12 Now complete the look by applying the remaining decals to your other toes.

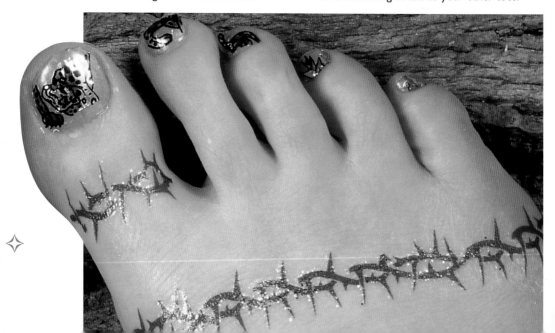

You Will Need

Base coat

Deep-purple nail enamel

Small pair of scissors

Cutout transfer

Bowl of water

Tweezers

Cotton bud

Rhinestones

Quick-drying clear topcoat

Gothic Twist

This design is made up of a combination of transfers and rhinestones. Depending on the color nail enamel that you use, you can create either a dramatic, Gothic appearance or a softer, more romantic look.

1 Apply the base coat to all of your nails and then two coats of deep-purple nail enamel, allowing each coat to dry thoroughly.

2 Dampen the decals with a moist cotton bud and position on the nail.

3 Using tweezers, place the rhinestones on the main edges of the transfer.

4 Apply two coats of quick-drying topcoat, allowing the first to dry thoroughly before applying the second, and making sure that the brush does not drag over the design.

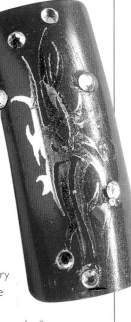

You Will Need

Base coat

Transfers

Small pair of scissors

Cotton bud

Container of water

Tweezers

Quick-drying clear topcoat

Bed of Roses

Another ultrafeminine design that will enhance a romantic evening.

1 Apply the base coat to each nail and allow it to dry.

2 Select the correct-size transfers and cut around the design so that each fits its designated nail. Place the decal face down in a container of water.

3 Using tweezers, carefully remove the transfer, position it over, and then slide it onto, your nail. Make sure that it is wrinkle-free by smoothing it with the damp cotton bud.

4 Gently brush an even layer of quick-drying topcoat over all of your nails.

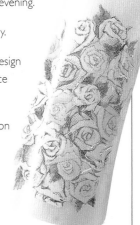

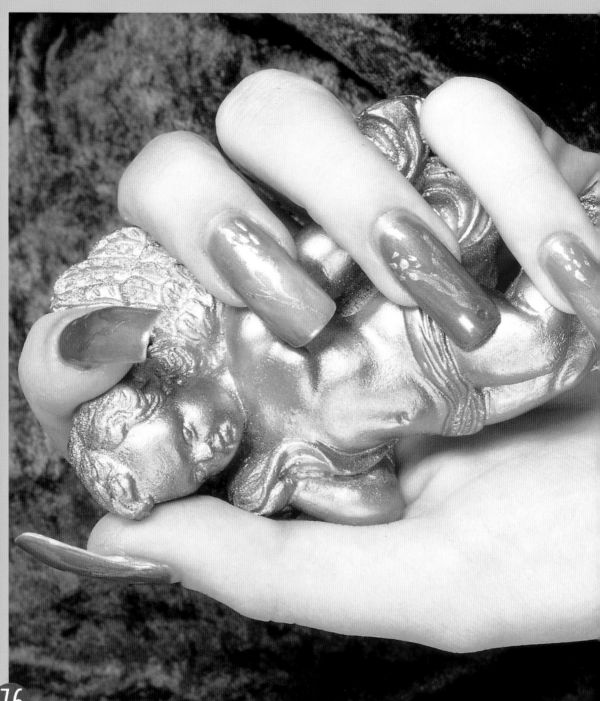

Freehand Nail Art

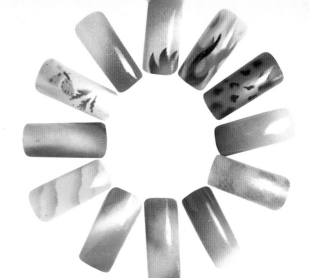

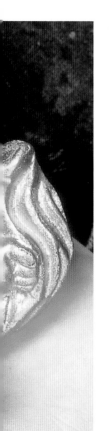

We have already seen how you can create beautiful and unusual nail designs using stick-on accessories and decals. However, for those with an adventurous heart and steady hand, you can achieve equally stunning effects with acrylic paints. You can apply these either with a fine-nibbed pen or a fine artist's brush (both available from art stores) dipped in a pot of your chosen color.

From simple line effects to flowers and swirling patterns, you can create any effect you desire. The following projects are just the beginning – once you've mastered the technique you can create stunning designs of your own. By combining freehand painting techniques with stick-on art, your nail style will be truly original!

It's often easier to work with friends to create designs on each others' nails, but the first project shows just how easy it is to decorate your own nails. The same techniques apply whether you are working on your own or someone else's nails. Remember to work slowly, and try to keep your hand as steady as possible.

Simple Coral

Thin, wavy lines are one of the easiest freehand patterns to achieve, and can look delicate or wild, depending on how many you paint – and how many colors you combine. Here we added some rhinestones for a glittering effect.

You Will Need

Base coat

True-red nail enamel

Fine-nibbed pen

Black acrylic paint

Silver acrylic paint

Tiny black and silver rhinestones

Orange stick
♦
Bowl of water
♦
Quick-drying clear topcoat

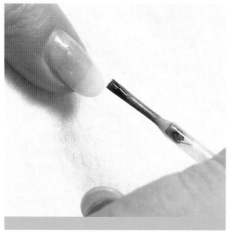

1 First apply the base coat to all of your nails.

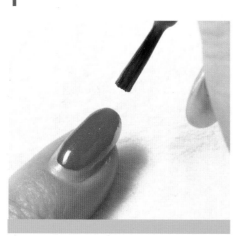

2 Then apply two coats of true-red enamel, allowing each coat to dry thoroughly.

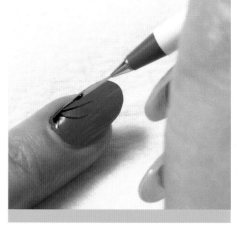

3 Using a fine-nibbed pen and black acrylic paint, paint a fine, wavy line at the side of your nail. Create a leaflike base with the point of your brush and then shade the motif completely.

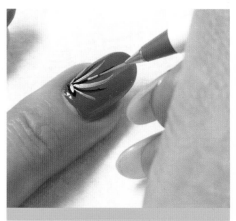

4 Following the same procedure, apply silver paint, using the finer pen to create slightly thinner and lighter strokes.

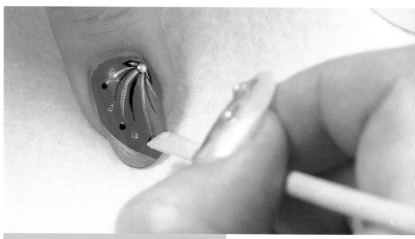

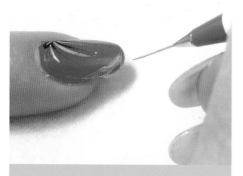

5 Apply a little silver paint to the tip of your nail for added shine.

6 Apply a little topcoat to your nail to secure the rhinestones. Using a dampened orange stick, carefully position the silver and black rhinestones. Finally, seal your design with a quick-drying top coat.

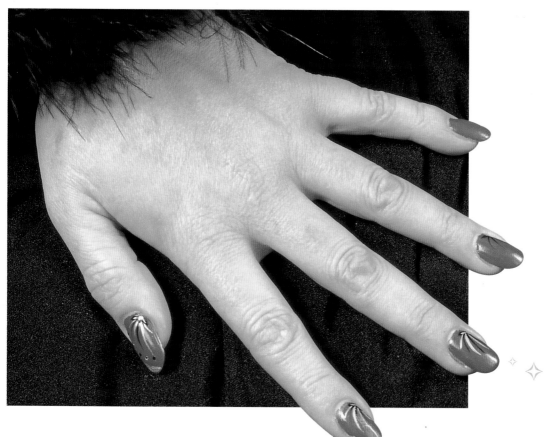

Flowers and Pearls

Here is a floral design that combines metallic paints with gold studs and pearls for a striking, but delicate, look.

You Will Need

Base coat

✧

True-clover
nail enamel

✧

Fine-nibbed pen

✧

Bronze acrylic paint

✧

Gold acrylic paint

✧

Orange stick

✧

Gold studs
(1 per nail)

✧

Pearls

✧

Bowl of water

✧

Quick-drying
clear topcoat

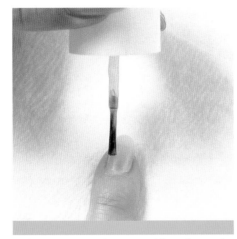

1 First apply your base coat. Allow this to dry thoroughly.

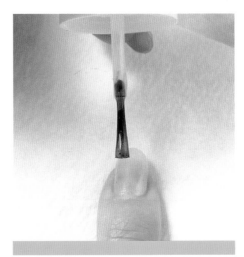

2 Then apply two coats of true-clover nail enamel to each nail. Allow each coat to dry thoroughly before continuing.

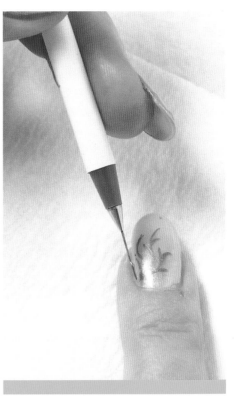

3 Using a fine-nibbed pen and bronze acrylic paint, use a loose, zigzagging motion to draw the stems.

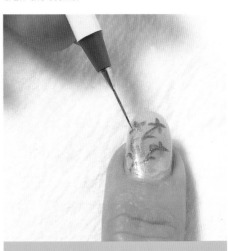

4 Create a four-leafed flower shape with the gold paint.

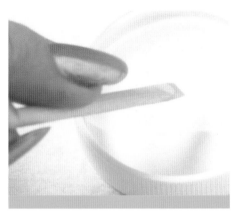

5 Apply some topcoat to the nail to act as a bonding agent. Using a dampened orange stick, pick up each gold stud in turn.

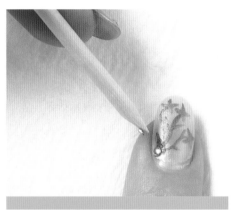

6 Place the gold studs on the tacky surface of the nail and then apply the pearls in the same way. Seal your design with a quick-drying topcoat.

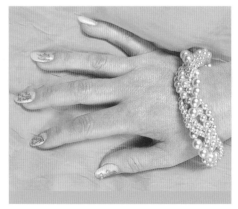

7 This is a design that works well either on one fingernail or across each nail.

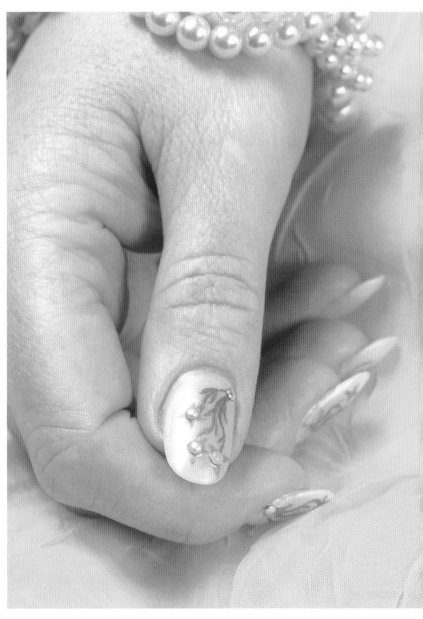

Royal Rococo

Gold, silver, and purple will add a
dramatic and decadent regal touch
to a special occasion.

You Will Need

Base coat

✧

Lilac nail enamel

✧

Medium-sized
art pen

✧

Gold acrylic paint

✧

Fine-nibbed pen

✧

Quick-drying
clear topcoat

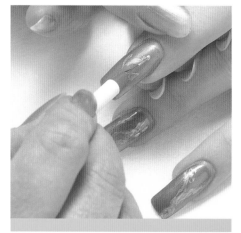

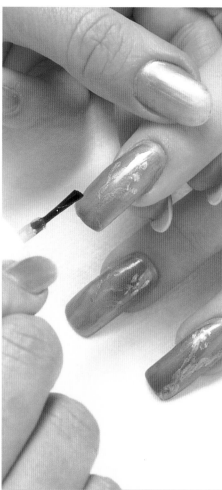

1 Apply a base coat and then two coats of
lilac enamel, allowing each to dry
completely. Use the medium-sized pen to
create a pattern of silver and gold dots.

3 Once you have completed the design, seal it
with a quick-drying topcoat.

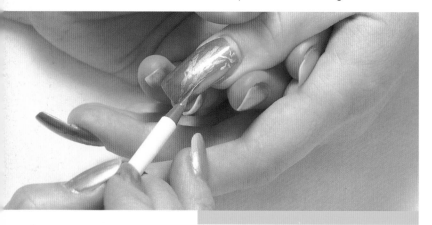

2 Using the fine-nibbed pen, make quick,
upward and outward strokes in a flicking
motion.

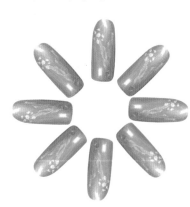

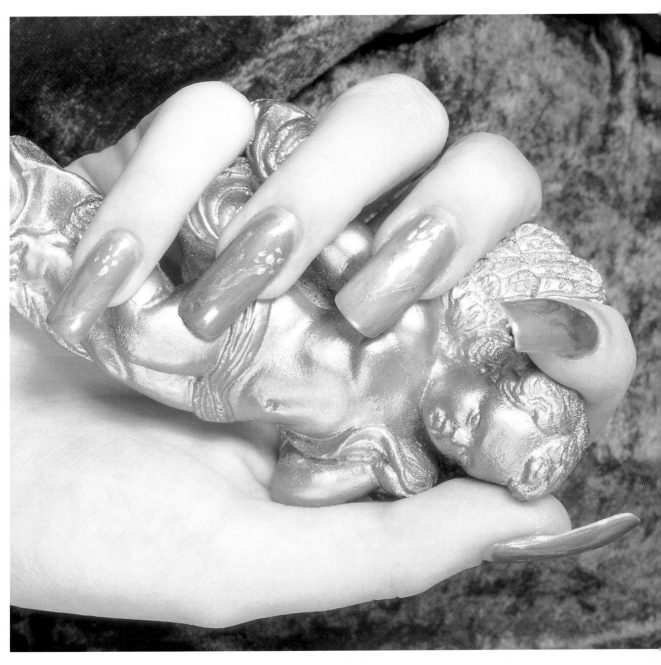

Simple Flower

The same painting techniques can be applied to false acrylic nails. This is ideal if you're worried about painting with a nail in place. Simply wait for the paint to dry and then apply the false nails (see page 93 for instructions).

You Will Need

Acrylic nail, prepainted with a color of your choice

✧

Medium-sized brush

✧

Acrylic paints

✧

Small brush

✧

Quick-drying clear topcoat

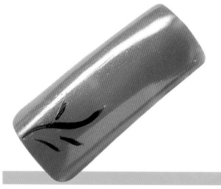

1 Using a medium-sized brush loaded with acrylic paint, touch the brush on your nail before pulling it down and then lifting it quickly in a jolting motion to achieve tapered ends.

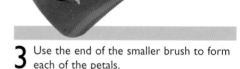

3 Use the end of the smaller brush to form each of the petals.

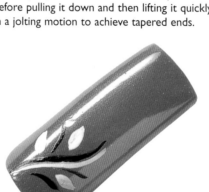

2 Use the smaller brush to paint the leaves in white and to add shading to the stem. Touch the brush on the nail and allow the bristles to spread so that they fill the designated area. Pull the brush downward and upward as you finish, so that you form a point.

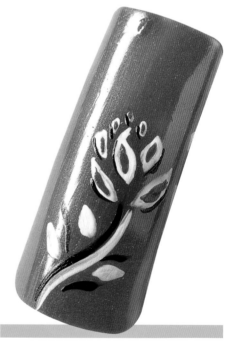

4 Paint small areas with one or more contrasting colors to give depth to your flower. Finally, apply a quick-drying topcoat to cover your design.

84

Psychedelic Dream

Opalescent paints can also be used to create a wilder, more random pattern. The effect looks best on a dark base, and you can paint on as many different colors as you wish.

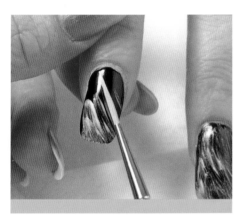

1 After applying base coat and two coats of your chosen topcoat, simply apply lines and swirls of opalescent paint to the nail. Use different-sized nibs for different effects, and build up a range of contrasting – or complementary – colors. Then seal with a topcoat to finish.

You Will Need

Base coat

✧

Dark-colored nail enamel

✧

Art pens – any-sized nib

✧

Acrylic paints – any color(s)

✧

Quick-drying clear topcoat

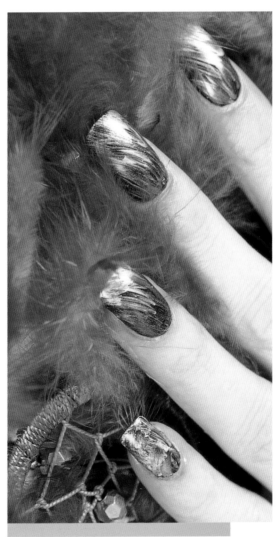

2 This is an excellent effect for an over-the-top party appearance!

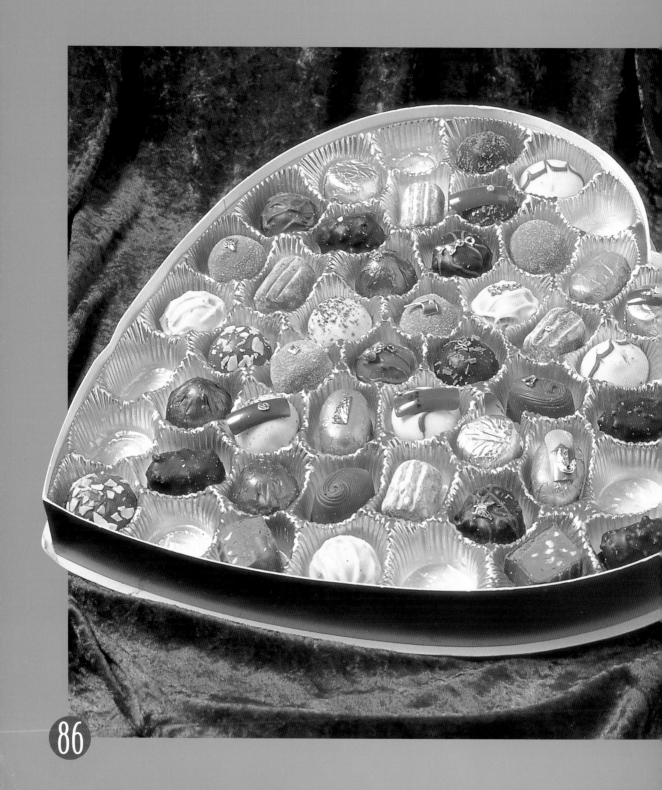

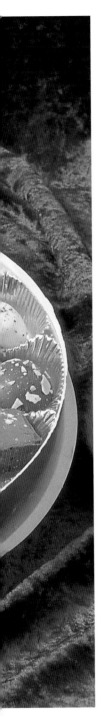

Advanced Nail Art

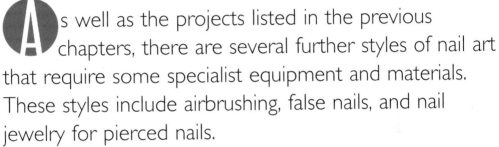

As well as the projects listed in the previous chapters, there are several further styles of nail art that require some specialist equipment and materials. These styles include airbrushing, false nails, and nail jewelry for pierced nails.

An airbrush enables you to spray a very fine mist of water-based paint onto your nail, creating shaded effects from two to three tones, depending on your creativity. The paint dries very quickly once you get into a routine spraying action. Always remember to apply at least two coats of base coat, both to protect your nail and to provide a canvas surface for your airbrushing.

Various kits exist for false acrylic nails, and some are more effective than others. They are a fun – and easy – way to brighten up your nails, and as long as you apply and remove them correctly, your own nails will not be damaged.

Piercing your nails can be tricky, and is probably best left to the professionals, as there is the risk that you may damage your nails. However, it is an effective, and safer technique to use on false nails.

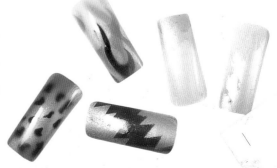

Airbrushing

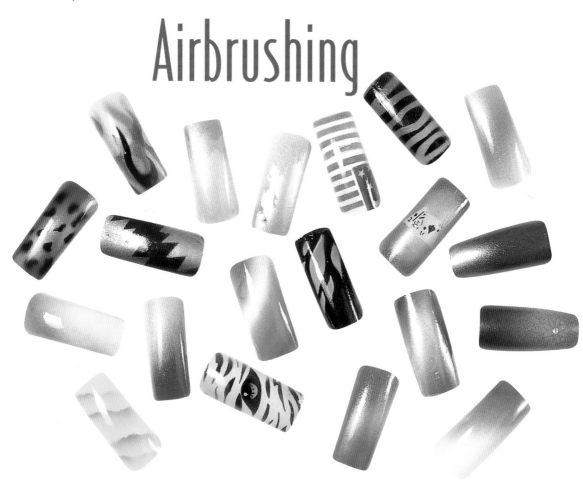

There are many different styles that can be achieved with airbrushing.

You can buy airbrushing kits that have been especially designed for nails. These are usually single-action systems that are stocked by most good art stores. You will also need to use special airbrushing paints and tools, along with airbrushing cleaners. (It is important that you keep your airbrush clean, because dried paint can clog it up, making producing airbrushed designs for your nails an extremely messy and frustrating process.)

The acrylic paints used with an airbrush are water-based and nontoxic, and can be bought in various dilutions, either premixed or you can mix them yourself. As well as standard colors, they are available in opalescent or neon colors.

You Will Need

Base coat

✧

Airbrushing
equipment

✧

Airbrush cleaner

✧

White, jade, and gold
airbrush paint

✧

Quick-drying clear
topcoat

Touch of the Irish

A delicate touch of gold brings some
sparkle to your nail tips.

1 Apply a basecoat, then spray your whole
nail with the white paint. Clean the airbrush
and fill it with the jade paint.

2 Spraying lightly in diagonal bands
across the nail, slowly build up the density
of the color. Clean your airbrush again.

3 Using the gold paint, spray lightly over the
tip to give a finished look.

4 Finally, seal with a topcoat.

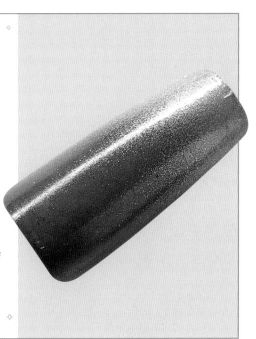

Tropical Haze

A tangy citrus look – ideal for summer.

1 Apply the base coat, allow it to dry, and then spray your nail white.

2 Clean the airbrush and spray the yellow across the nail in diagonal
bands, building up the density of the color and shading it into light.

3 Having cleaned the airbrush, spray the orange paint, diagonally across the
center of your nail, spraying lightly to build up the color as before.

4 After cleaning the airbrush, spray the lime green
diagonally to finish the striped pattern.. Seal with topcoat.

You Will Need

Base coat

✧

Airbrushing equipment

✧

Airbrush cleaner

✧

White, lime green,
orange, and yellow
airbrush paint

✧

Quick-drying clear
topcoat

89

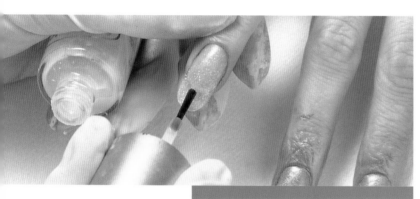

Nail Style
Goldfinger

A truly eye-catching design! The gold hand effect shown here is simply to highlight the dramatic appearance of the nails – we don't recommend that you try to repeat this loo, unless you're off to a fancy-dress party – even then, apply paint minimally to your skin and for a short time only.

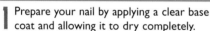

You Will Need

Base coat
✦
Airbrushing equipment
✦
Airbrush cleaner
✦
White, gold, and orange paint
✦
Quick-drying clear topcoat

1 Prepare your nail by applying a clear base coat and allowing it to dry completely.

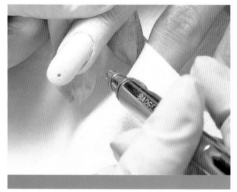

3 Apply white paint over the entire nail, from the tip into the center of the nail. Make sure that your airbrush is spraying an even and light spray.

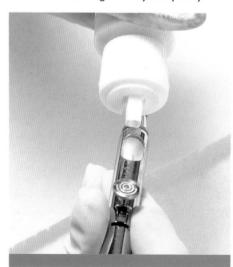

2 Now fill the airbrush with the white paint. This is sprayed over the entire nail to obtain the maximum clarity of color shading and definition.

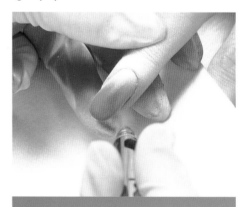

4 Clean the airbrush and fill it with orange paint Apply this to nail in the same way as in step 3. To give more density, spray fine layers of paint by moving the airbrush slowly backward and forward, building up layers; for paler shading, spray more lightly.

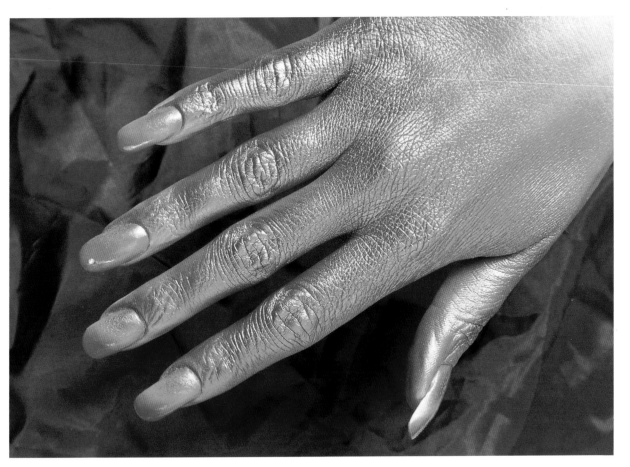

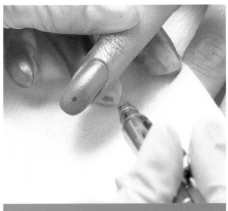

5 Now apply the gold paint. It is very important that you keep your airbrush clean at all times. A clogged airbrush will spit out paint and spoil the smooth effect.

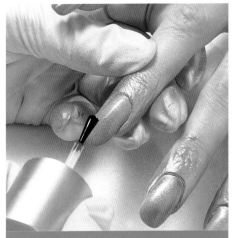

6 Finally, seal with a topcoat.

91

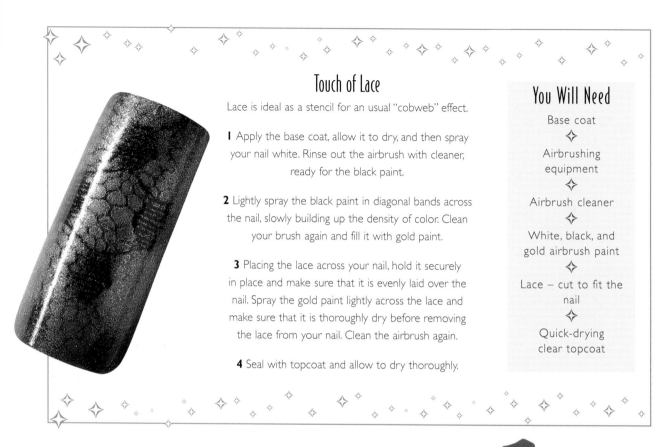

Touch of Lace

Lace is ideal as a stencil for an usual "cobweb" effect.

1 Apply the base coat, allow it to dry, and then spray your nail white. Rinse out the airbrush with cleaner, ready for the black paint.

2 Lightly spray the black paint in diagonal bands across the nail, slowly building up the density of color. Clean your brush again and fill it with gold paint.

3 Placing the lace across your nail, hold it securely in place and make sure that it is evenly laid over the nail. Spray the gold paint lightly across the lace and make sure that it is thoroughly dry before removing the lace from your nail. Clean the airbrush again.

4 Seal with topcoat and allow to dry thoroughly.

You Will Need

Base coat

✧

Airbrushing equipment

✧

Airbrush cleaner

✧

White, black, and gold airbrush paint

✧

Lace – cut to fit the nail

✧

Quick-drying clear topcoat

Chevron Extension

This is a quick and easy way to achieve an interesting variation on a traditional French polish. Apply the nail extensions according to the instructions given in the first project. This look is perfect for romantic occasions.

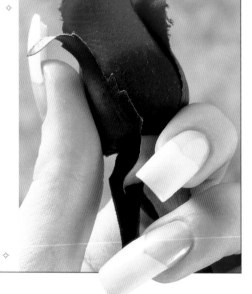

Extensions and Stick-on Nails

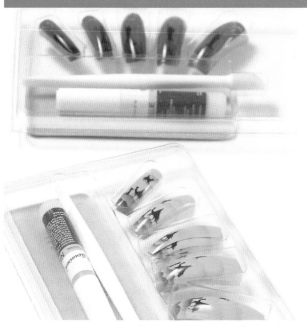

Stick-on nails can be bought in packs or applied by a qualified technician.

Extensions are available in many shapes, designs, and forms, including airbrushed patterns, French polish, square-finished, or curved-tipped, and are normally secured with two forms of adhesive, either double-sided sticky-back or nail glue. They cover the entire nail plate and it is necessary to size up each nail individually before securing them.

Extensions can be cut to any length, from very short and neat to wickedly long. They provide a fantastic canvas for nail art. Decorated nail extensions can be bought, but vary in quality. You may need to visit a professional nail technician for a finished look.

Glittering Acrylics

Here, shapes have been cut out of a nail extension and a clear acrylic nail tip fastened on top. Again, this uses the same technique as described in the first project (page 32). For a fabulous party look, a coat of holographic acrylic glitter enamel has been applied over the top, which shows up wonderfully under pulsing disco lights!

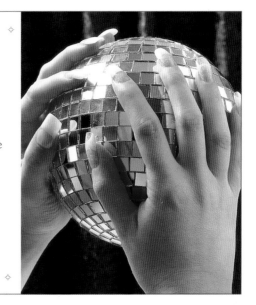

Tropical Sunset

You Will Need

Orange stick

✧

Acetone-free nail-
enamel remover

✧

Emery board

✧

Stick-on nail-
extension kit

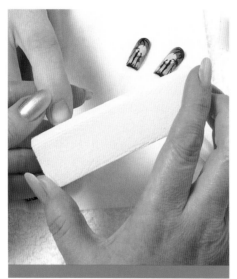

1 Remove any existing nail enamel or grease
that may create a film over your natural
nail. Gently push your cuticles back using an
orange stick wrapped in absorbent cotton
and buff your nails.

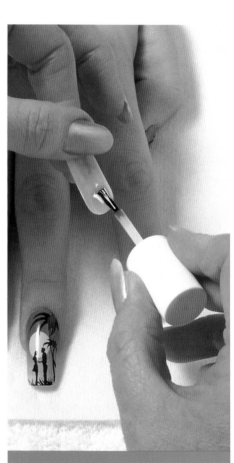

3 Pierce the top of the glue (from the kit)
and apply a small amount over the length of
your nail tip.

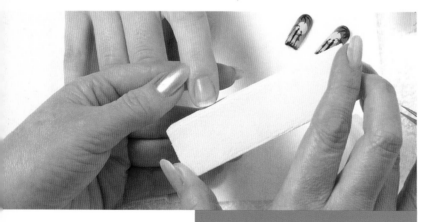

2 Align the false nail over your natural nail
for the best fit. If you need to file the nail,
take care not to damage the design or
decoration. Once you have done this, lay out
all ten nails in order for ease of use.

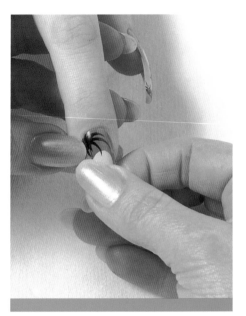

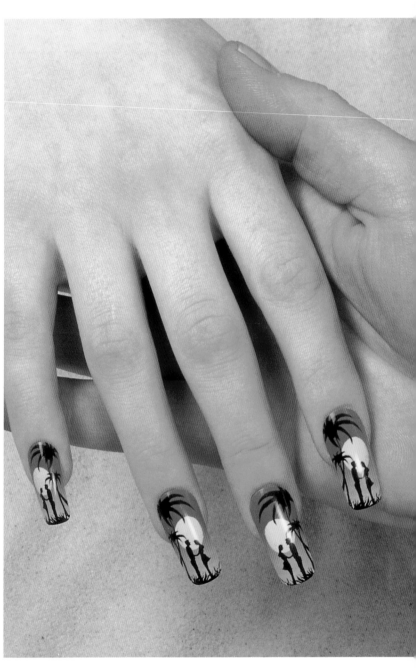

4 Hold the nail tip at a slight angle, place the end into the cuticle area of the natural nail, and slowly, but firmly, lower it onto your natural nail. Always try to make sure that you check that it is secure by looking down along the nail (end on) to ensure that there are no gaps, as these can create air pockets which could cause the false nail to come off.

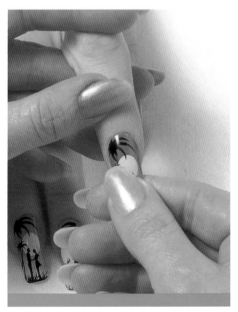

5 Allow the glue 30 seconds to set and then continue with the other nails.

Nail Jewelry

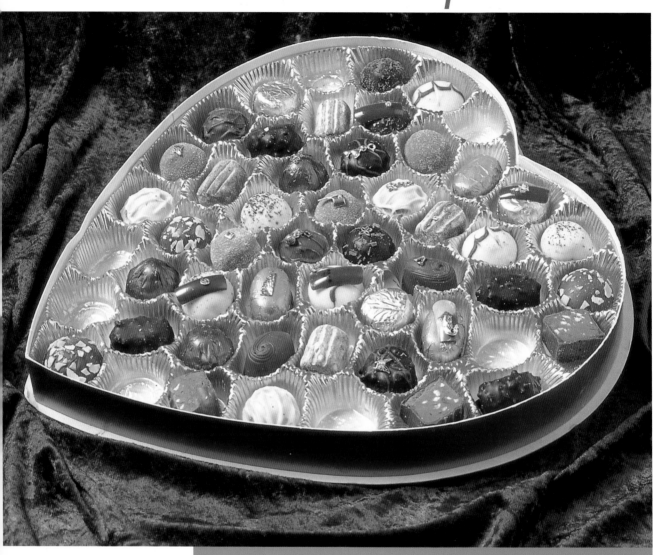

Nail jewelry can be truly "sweet" temptation!

Nail jewelry can complement any form of nail art, from the most subtle to the most outrageous. It comes in many forms, from simple, clip-on jewelry through full-posted charms or scrolls, to diamonds that are linked by a chain to a ring on your finger. Gold, silver, copper, or platinum nail tips, which are often engraved with designs and studded with gems, can also include chains incorporated into a ring.

Sometimes you will have to pierce your nail to hold nail jewelry in place. If you wish to pierce your own nail, it is vital that you protect it with a layer of durable acrylic (do not use fiberglass or gel). The reason why the nail must be protected is that the structure of the nail will otherwise be weakened: once it has been pierced it can lose strength from its center core and collapse at the edges. It is essential that a qualified nail technician coats the nail with acrylic, after which you can cut the nail to any length you want. You can then safely invest in any number of nail-jewelry kits, which will usually supply you with a charm and drill. For this reason, we are using false acrylic nails to demonstrate the technique.

Clip-on nail jewelry is attached with a jump ring, but the jump ring is usually not wide enough to reach the center of the nail. Diamonds or full pieces of nail jewelry and design need to be more securely attached and balanced. Remember that if you want to place a diamond in the center of your nail, you will need to pierce the nail slightly off center. In the case of clip-on nail art, make sure that you pierce your nail closer to the side walls and outer edge, and not too close to the free edge, so that your nail and jewelry retain balance and stability.

For pierced nail jewelry, you will need a small combidrill. These can be readily obtained from beauty parlors or arts and crafts suppliers. If in doubt, ask a professional nail technician for advice. It is essential that you keep your hand steady when drilling, so you will also need a finger rest or nail-support buffer.

Warning!

If you drill the hole in the wrong place, perhaps too close to the free edge or tip of your nail, you could not only damage the nail plate, but could also break the nail, especially if the charm is heavy. These are further reasons why you should always make sure that your nail has been coated with acrylic before drilling it.

All of the following projects require that you attach a false acrylic nail to the finger(s) you wish to adorn. For instructions on applying false nails, see page 94.

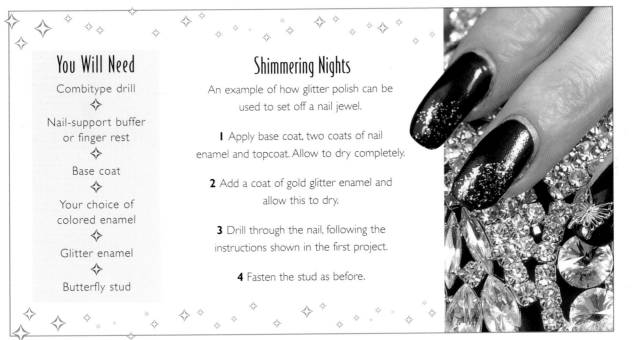

You Will Need

Combitype drill

✧

Nail-support buffer or finger rest

✧

Base coat

✧

Your choice of colored enamel

✧

Glitter enamel

✧

Butterfly stud

Shimmering Nights

An example of how glitter polish can be used to set off a nail jewel.

1 Apply base coat, two coats of nail enamel and topcoat. Allow to dry completely.

2 Add a coat of gold glitter enamel and allow this to dry.

3 Drill through the nail, following the instructions shown in the first project.

4 Fasten the stud as before.

Diamonds are Forever

A diamond charm is one of the most popular pieces of nail jewelry, and can be used to decorate any of your fingers. It can also add a dramatic look to a number of nail-art designs. The diamonds usually come in two styles: bezel or claw (a bezel gives the smoothest finish). Remember not to attempt this project until you have had your nail coated with acrylic by a professional.

You Will Need

Combitype drill
✧
Nail-support buffer
or finger rest
✧
Base coat
✧
Black enamel
✧
Post-ended
diamond charm

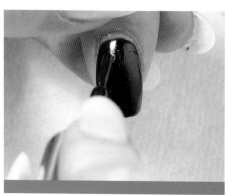

1 Apply a base coat and two coats of black nail enamel. Allow to dry thoroughly.

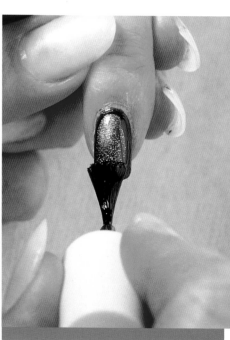

3 Finally apply a clear topcoat, again, allowing it to dry completely.

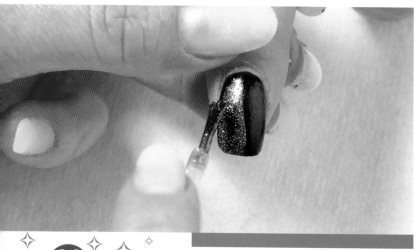

2 Add a coat of silver glitter enamel. This will complement the effect of the diamond stud. Allow to dry.

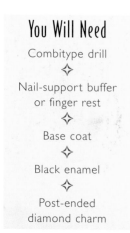

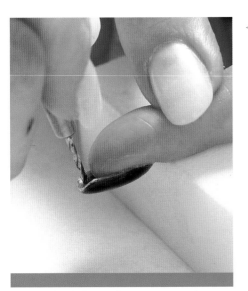

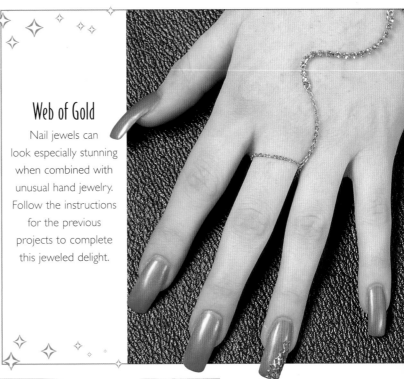

Web of Gold

Nail jewels can look especially stunning when combined with unusual hand jewelry. Follow the instructions for the previous projects to complete this jeweled delight.

4 Rest the drill on a finger rest or nail-support buffer and position the tip approximately 3mm (1/8") from the nail tip. First drill from the back of the nail. Turning the drill several times, carefully apply enough pressure to pierce the nail.

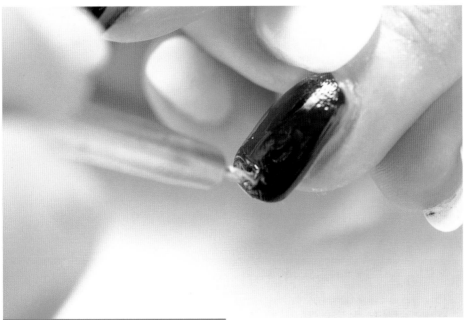

5 Now turn your hand over and redrill from the front of the nail.

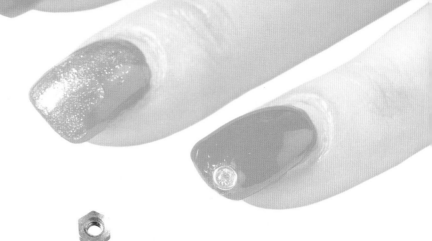

6 Separate the jewel from the stud and slide the post of the jewel through the pierced hole. Be careful not to scratch the polish.

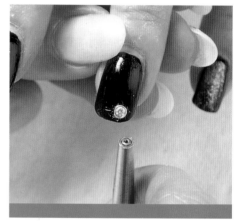

8 Fasten the stud to the back of the jewel by turning the bolt to secure the charm.

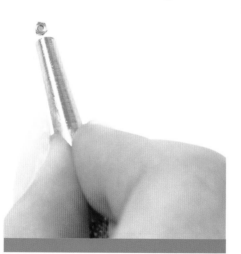

7 Using the other end of the drill bit, place the nut in the open end of the drill bit supporting the diamond charm and place the socket end of the drill on the post-ended charm stem.

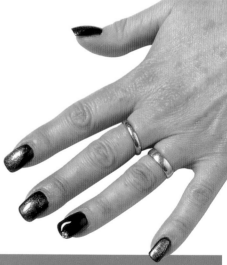

9 This is a particularly stunning effect when the other nails are left plain.

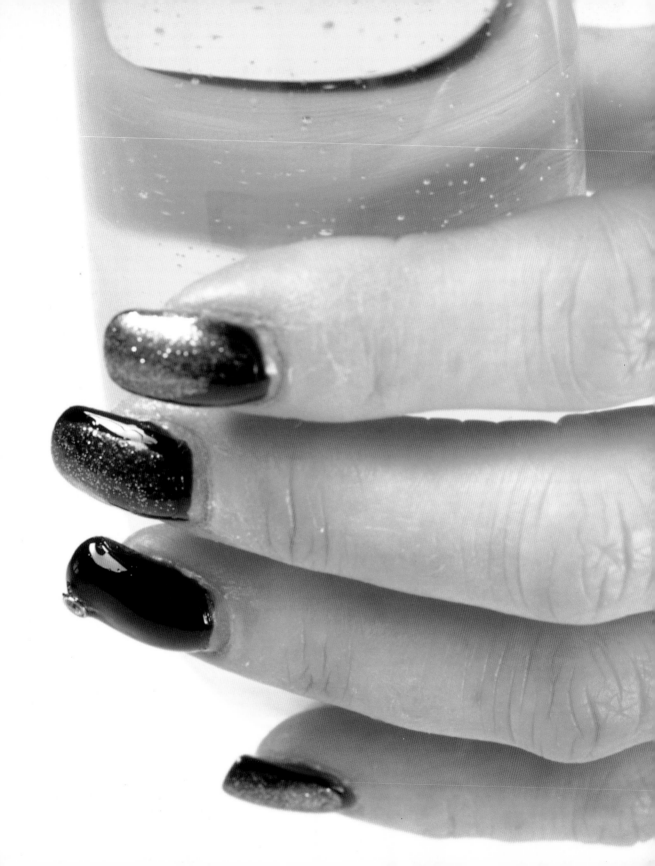

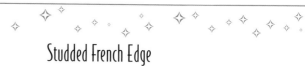

Studded French Edge

Most nail tips look the most attractive on a ring or little finger, but the choice is yours.

You Will Need

White block (soft)	Cotton bud
✦	✦
Professional nail glue	Acetone nail-enamel remover
✦	✦
1 x 14 carat gold nail	1 x soft paper tissue

1 Make sure that your nail is clean and free of oil or nail enamel.

2 To ensure maximum bonding, gently buff your nail with a soft white block (see page 27).

3 Carefully apply a small amount of nail glue to your nail
(remember that it is a fast-drying bonding agent).

4 Positioning it at an angle, place the end of the gold nail on the edge of your cuticle. Slowly lower it over your nail and then hold it firmly in place for approximately 10 to 15 seconds.

5 If you have been over-generous with the bonding agent, you may
have to remove some excess nail glue from around the edge of the nail.
Use a cotton bud dampened with acetone nail-enamel remover.

6 Buff your new nail with a soft paper tissue.

Teardrop

Ring-clip charms are usually placed on the inner or outer edge of the tip of your nail. Remember not to attempt this project until you have had your nail coated with acrylic by a professional. You may also prefer them to pierce your nail for you.

You Will Need

Combitype drill
✧
Nail-support buffer or finger rest
✧
Base coat
✧
Your choice of colored enamel
✧
Chain ring-clip and nail jewelry

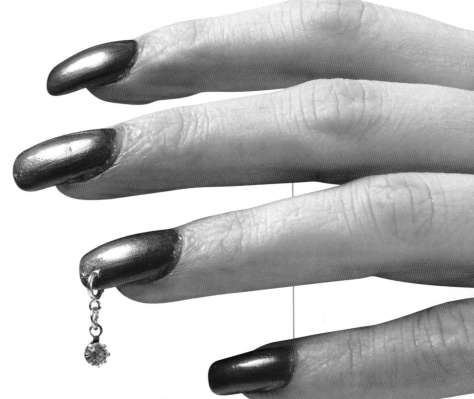

1 If you wish to drill your own nail, position the drill tip approximately 3mm (1/8") from the tip of your nail. Supporting the drill on a nail-support buffer or finger rest, slowly revolve it to the right, using a circular movement, until you can feel it touch the buffer or nail support.

2 Pull down the trigger on the ring clip to open the clasp (like a jump ring on a chain). Making sure that the trigger doesn't catch on your nail, insert it in the hole on the underside of the nail.

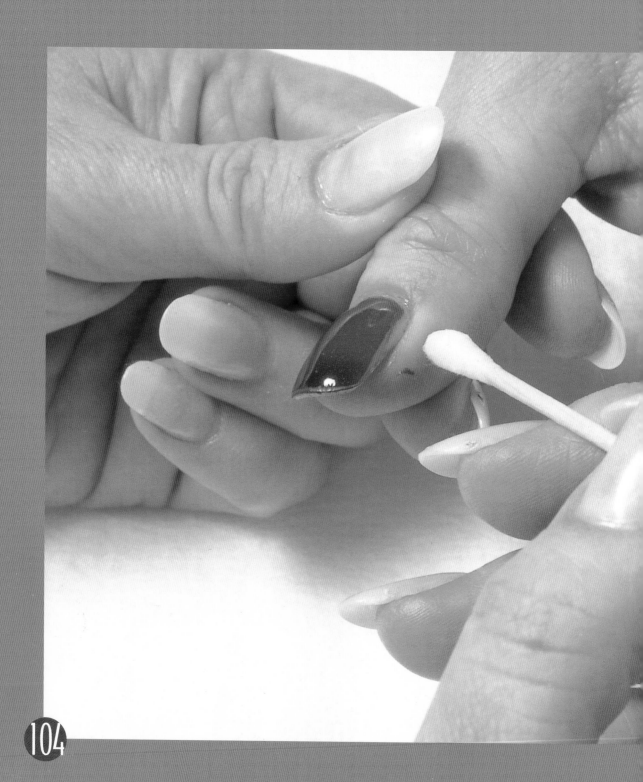

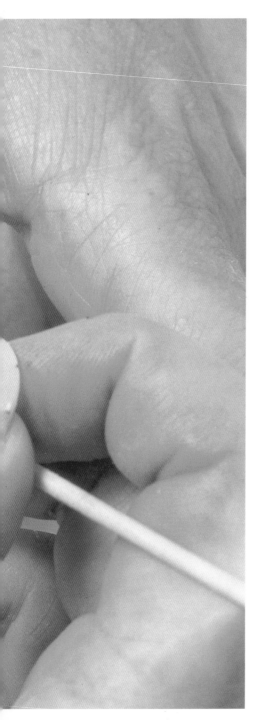

Here Today, Gone Tomorrow

Most nail art, whether an enamel, decals, or false nails, is simple to remove. Always make sure that you follow the instructions carefully, as you can cause damage if you try to remove decorative effects in haste, or with the wrong removing agent.

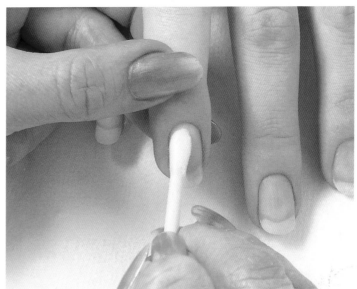

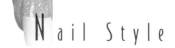
Removal and Aftercare

It is essential that you always remove nail art or nail enamel and follow this with a natural manicure. Good-quality nail jewelry is reusable, so clean it thoroughly after each use.

Removing Nail Enamel

Before removing your nail enamel, make sure that you have some acetone-free nail-enamel remover and a cotton pad or absorbent cotton to hand.

Pour a generous amount of nail-enamel remover on to the cotton pad and then press the pad on to your nail for a few seconds to achieve maximum saturation. Drag the pad toward you firmly, using a right-to-left motion (this will ensure that you do not cover your entire finger with the dissolved enamel, which can make a horrible mess, especially in the case of bright-red or dark-colored enamels).

Once you have removed the enamel, remember to wash your hands, because any remaining nail-enamel remover can dehydrate your nails. If some enamel remains around the edges of your nails, clean it off with an orange stick or cotton pad. Finally, if you are not going to repaint your nails immediately, always apply a good-quality hand cream.

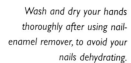

Use an orange stick to clean away any remaining nail enamel.

Wash and dry your hands thoroughly after using nail-enamel remover, to avoid your nails dehydrating.

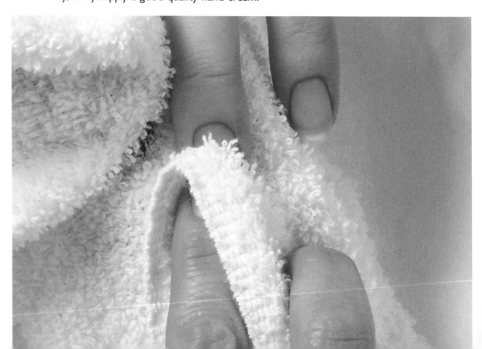

Removing Nail Art

Remember to allow plenty of time when removing nail art, as this is not a five-minute job. If you are wearing clip-on nail jewelry, always take it off and store it safely before removing your nail art. You may sometimes have to wash your nail jewelry, in which case do so gently, perhaps using a specialized jewelry-cleaning product.

Following the same procedure as for the removal of nail enamel (see above), remove each layer of your nail-art design with an acetone-free nail-enamel remover.

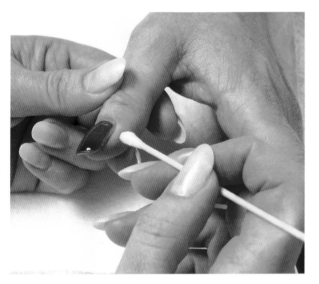

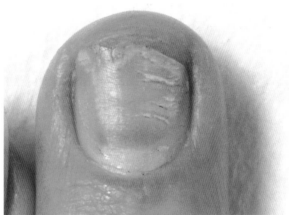

A cotton bud can also be used to remove excess enamel that has slipped onto your fingers after application.

Excessive use of false nails, or incorrect removal, can cause serious damage which will take a long time to heal. If in doubt, have false nails removed by a professional.

Removing False Nails

The method for removing stick-on nails varies according to which type you are wearing. Double-sided stick-on nails can be removed quite easily with an acetone-containing nail-enamel remover. Saturate a pad or ball of absorbent cotton with the nail-enamel remover, hold it firmly over the false nail for a few seconds, and then gently rotate the pad to break down the false nail. In the case of stubborn glue, pour a glue solvent onto a cotton bud and gently rub it over your nail to break down the glue.

Always wash your hands thoroughly after removing stick-on nails. You should ideally have allowed enough time to give yourself a manicure, but if you are in a hurry, apply nail moisturizer and hand cream instead.

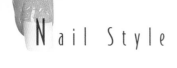

Removing Nail Extensions

The removal method will vary according to the type of nail extension, be it fiberglass, gel, or acrylic. It is usually best done by a qualified nail technician, but kits are available to buy. If you have bought a removal kit, make sure that you follow the instructions to the letter and that you apply an intensive hand cream after you have completed your manicure.

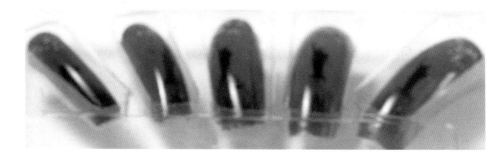

Removing Bonded Nail Jewelry

Remove bonded nail jewelry, such as a gold nail tip, with a bonding remover. First dot a few drops of bonding remover all around the cuticle and free edge of your nail. Massage it in gently to help loosen the jewelry (it can often take 10 to 15 minutes to soften the bonding agent). Carefully remove the nail jewelry and then wipe your nail with a damp cotton pad or cotton bud soaked in acetone nail-enamel remover to remove any residue. Apply a little cuticle oil, wash your hands, and then gently buff your nail with a white glass block.

The number of times that you can remove your nail jewelry without causing damage or discoloration and then reuse it depends on its quality.

Index

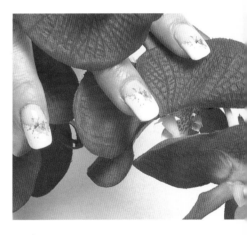

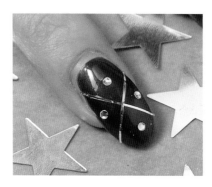

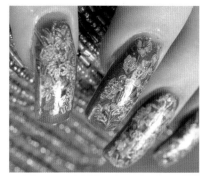
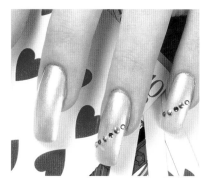

Credits and Acknowledgements

The author and publishers would like to thank the models for their patience and dedication:

Marc Bowers
Suzanne Crick
Shelley Dockery-Turner
Tina Jopling

Additional thanks to:

Jason Shaw from N.S.I. for his help and support.
EzFlow for their designer glittering acrylics.
Karen for help with freehand designs.
Tina for her assistance in writing the book.

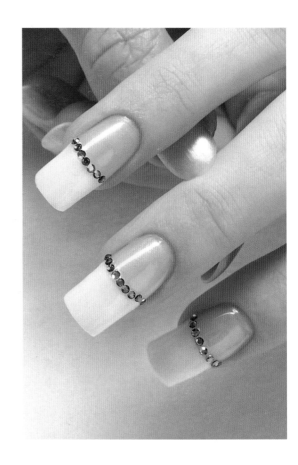